Complications of Cardiopulmonary Surgery

Other Volumes in This Series

Complications of Surgery in General
J. A. R. Smith

Complications of Minor Surgery
C. J. Stoddard and J. A. R. Smith

Complications of Total Joint Replacement
N. Kay

Complications of Urology and Transplant Surgery
R. F. M. Wood and M. C. Bishop

Complications of Surgical Oncology
R. D. Rosin

Complications of Paediatric Surgery
J. Lister

Complications in the Management of Breast Disease
R. W. Blamey

Complications of Biliary and Pancreatic Surgery
C. W. Imrie

Complications of Arterial Surgery
R. Baird

Complications of Endocrine Surgery
I. D. A. Johnston

Complications of Surgery of the Hand
S. Norris

Complications of Spinal Surgery
R. A. Dickson and M. Cameron

Complications of Gynaecological Oncology
J. Monaghan

Complications of Plastic Surgery
A. M. Morris, A. C. H. Watson and J. H. Stevenson

Complications of Surgery of the Lower Gastrointestinal Tract
I. Taylor and J. A. R. Smith

Complications of Surgery of the Upper Gastrointestinal Tract
R. M. Kirk and C. J. Stoddard

Complications in Surgery
Edited by John A. R. Smith

Complications of Cardiopulmonary Surgery

Geoffrey H. Smith
MB, BS, FRCS

Consultant Cardiothoracic Surgeon, Northern General Hospital, Sheffield; Honorary Clinical Lecturer, Department of Cardiothoracic Surgery, University of Sheffield

Baillière Tindall London Philadelphia Toronto
Mexico City Rio de Janeiro Sydney Tokyo Hong Kong

Baillière Tindall 1 St Anne's Road
W. B. Saunders Eastbourne, East Sussex BN21 3UN, England

West Washington Square
Philadelphia, PA 19105, USA

1 Goldthorne Avenue
Toronto, Ontario M8Z 5T9, Canada

Apartado 26370—Cedro 512
Mexico 4, DF, Mexico

Rua Evaristo da Veiga 55, 20° andar
Rio de Janeiro—RJ, Brazil

ABP Australia Ltd, 44 Waterloo Road
North Ryde, NSW 2113, Australia

Ichibancho Central Building, 22-1 Ichibancho
Chiyoda-ku, Tokyo 102, Japan

10/FL, Inter-Continental Plaza, 94 Granville Road
Tsim Sha Tsui East, Kowloon, Hong Kong

First published 1984

Printed in Great Britain at the Alden Press, Oxford

British Library Cataloguing in Publication Data

Smith, Geoffrey H.
Complications of cardiopulmonary surgery.
—(Complications in surgery)
1. Chest—Surgery—Complications and sequelae
I. Title II. Series
617'.5401 RD536

ISBN 0-7020-1050-2

Contents

Series Foreword

All doctors who are involved in the care of surgical patients are all too aware of the hazards of the operation and the morbidity and mortality that can result from an ill considered or ill managed procedure, and of the complications, whether related directly to the operation, the disease process, the patient or even to the hospital environment. It is also true to say that many hospitals are now mindful of these difficulties and have introduced a pattern of regular medical audit through which the extent and the significance of the problem can be identified and which, when necessary, can point to the remedy.

The majority of complications are of course preventable by careful preoperative preparation, by skilled operative technique and by proper postoperative care, but when they do occur, it is the early recognition, the immediate and correct investigation, and the awareness of the operative treatment that will decide the eventual outcome and the likelihood of early recovery.

Obviously every surgeon would like to believe that in his own practice complications will be, at the least, occasional events and hopefully this is the case in most hospitals. The corollary of this is, however, that the personal experience of many surgeons in these serious potential or actual problems is not great and the opportunities for the trainee surgeon to learn about them, and about their clinical significance and management, are less than adequate.

This deficiency of experience in the average surgeon, whether general surgeon or specialist, has now been appreciated and John Smith in this series of texts has set out to provide what has been termed a 'reference point' from which the surgeon will be able to increase his awareness of the problems and increase his knowledge in areas where he is unlikely to gain experience from clinical practice. The prime aim of the series has been to ensure that knowledge of the existence of complications increases, that prevention can become more widely accepted and that the recognition and management of established complications can be undertaken with skill and competence.

Each of the volumes in the series considers a specific area of surgical practice and, in each, authorities in the field have presented their experience and their views in such a way that it will not only instruct but will also stimulate the reader to study the subject further.

It is undoubtedly an area of surgical practice that is of major importance and which has been somewhat neglected in the past. This is the first time that there has been an attempt to present a comprehensive account covering all aspects of practice and it will undoubtedly be a significant contribution to patient care in its broadest interpretation.

Sir James Fraser Bt, PRCS(Ed)
Nicolson Street
Edinburgh

Editor's foreword

Most textbooks of surgery acknowledge that postoperative complications exist and some describe methods of prevention or options for their further management. However, it is clear to me from conversations with junior staff, candidates for higher degrees and trainees in all branches of surgery that there is no reference to which they can turn where the complex problem of complications is adequately considered, i.e. covering details of aetiology, predisposition and methods of prevention, together with advice on which complications are likely to be encountered and how they may be recognized, investigated and managed.

This series is directed at all surgical trainees and also at the consultant working outside specialist referral centres. The latter may not often encounter the complications which are under consideration, but when they are encountered the surgeon needs advice on what to do, what not to do and, finally, when specialist referral is indicated.

The authors in this series are all consultants with a specialist practice in teaching hospitals. Each has been asked to provide the necessary information and to be dogmatic where that is possible, but to advise on the options where the situation is less clear. Points of persisting controversy have been identified.

The multi-authored text has been avoided, specifically to preclude confusion through differences of opinion within an individual volume. Each volume is self-sufficient, except that *Complications of Surgery in General* deals with all general surgical complications to avoid detailed repetition in the other, more specialist, volumes. Inevitably there is some overlap between volumes but I feel this to be preferable to omitting topics that may be important. Detailed references have not been included as a deliberate policy of the series, but suggestions for further reading are provided.

Finally, not all the complications described have been created by the authors; the selection of topic reflects, rather, their ability to deal with such problems as are referred to them!

The concept of a single volume on *Complications in Surgery* arose from discussions involving, on separate occasions, Mrs Ann Saadi (lately of Baillière Tindall), Mr R.M. Kirk (Royal Free Hospital, London) and myself. The volume has grown into a series but acknowledgements are due to Mrs Saadi and Mr Kirk for the idea and to Mrs Saadi for the enthusiasm which ensured the launch. I am most grateful to Dr Geoffrey Smaldon of Baillière Tindall who has now assumed responsibility for the entire series and has encouraged or cajoled as necessary. The artistic talent of Mr Pat Elliott is clear for all to see and is greatly appreciated. Finally, I am happy to acknowledge the support and encouragement of my wife and family.

John A. R. Smith
University Surgical Unit
Royal Hallamshire Hospital
Sheffield

Preface

Most surgeons in training now spend some time in cardiothoracic surgery. This specialty, lying as it does in between the traditional areas of 'medicine' and 'surgery', creates a range of new problems for young surgeons who have been immersed in orthopaedic and abdominal surgery. Familiarity with cardiac and respiratory drugs is needed and even the plain chest X-ray and electrocardiograph will cause problems.

In addition, cardiothoracic surgery is no longer a unified specialty. The surgery of the oesophagus is evolving as a separate specialty in the same way as the surgery of congenital heart disease before it. It is for these reasons that this volume concentrates on the cardiac and pulmonary problems – oesophageal and tracheal surgery are dealt with in another volume in this series.

This book is designed to appeal to those trainee surgeons coming into cardiothoracic surgery for a limited period in their training. I hope the book will also be used by those surgeons beginning to prepare for specialty examinations, such as the Fellowship in Edinburgh, and by those truly general surgeons working in areas remote from a cardiothoracic centre who meet problems within the chest occasionally. The book will not satisfy the trained, or nearly trained, cardiothoracic surgeon and will be too advanced for undergraduates.

Any surgeon writing of complications does so with very mixed feelings. Complications in cardiothoracic surgery involve all the members of the surgical and intensive care ward team. The support and encouragement given by the various members of that team is one of the attractions of the specialty and I wish to thank all those with whom I have gained the experience necessary to write this book.

Mr Pat Elliott, Medical Illustrator, and the Department of Medical Photography at the Northern General Hospital, Sheffield, have provided the illustrations and I give them thanks. My thanks also go to Miss Alison Ward for typing the manuscript and to Dr Geoffrey Smaldon of Baillière Tindall for his patience, skill and advice.

Finally, this book could not have been written without the help, criticism and unswerving support of my wife and daughters and I thank them.

Geoffrey H. Smith
1984

To Brenda,
my wife and best friend

1 Pain Control after Cardiothoracic Operations

All surgeons have the responsibility of controlling pain after patients have had an operation. Familiarity with the operations performed tends to make the surgeon minimize the degree of discomfort which every patient experiences after an operation. Non-medical people, however, are more realistic and most studies have shown that most patients expect considerable pain after surgery.

Adequate analgesia receives great attention after cardiothoracic operations, not because the operations are particularly painful as compared with other procedures but because anything other than adequate pain relief brings such immediate and obvious consequences. In addition, those looking after the patient tend to be very concerned about the possibility of respiratory depression. Inadequate pain control, therefore, causes severe complications which may be life threatening (see flow diagram overleaf). Every patient will have a personally unique level of pain threshold and the doctor has no way of determining this beforehand. Therefore, the analgesic requirements of each patient are also unique and independent of the type of operation performed. In addition, the patient with adequate constant pain control will be found to have a lower total analgesic requirement than one whose pain is allowed to go untreated from time to time.

Since pain is a subjective sensation, it therefore follows that the patient who complains of pain is, in fact, in need of analgesia. This plainly self-evident statement is often disregarded by those looking after the patient for a variety of reasons, including a lack of sympathy, worry about respiratory depression and an inadequate analgesic regimen. The patient who is in pain needs analgesia quickly and effectively, and provided that the total analgesic agent given just controls pain respiratory depression will not be produced.

Intravenous Analgesia

At the time of writing, pain is usually controlled by opiates such as morphine or papaveretum (Omnopon). Since the effect is

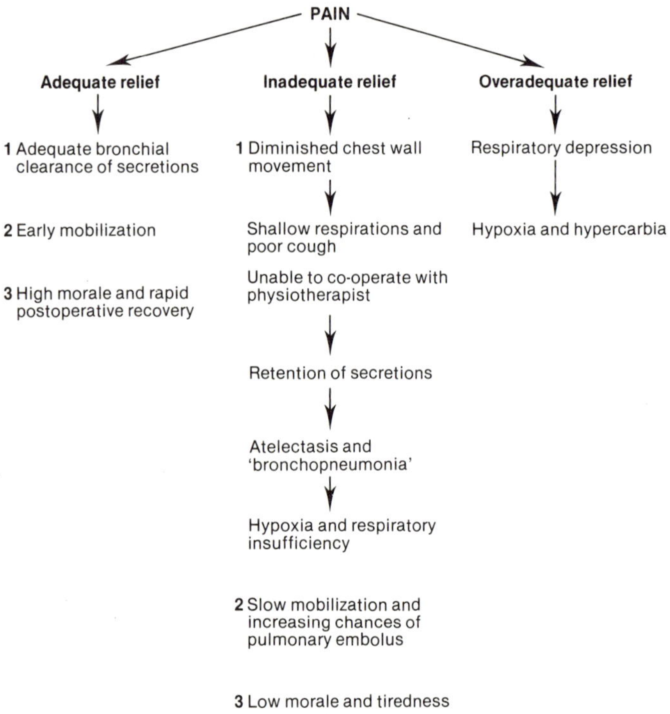

needed quickly, intravenous administration of small amounts (say papaveretum 5 mg) is given every five minutes until pain control is achieved. The amount which has to be given varies from patient to patient and sometimes 70 mg of papaveretum will be required for an adult. Intravenous injection means that the drug is rapidly absorbed and distributed with immediate effect. We have used this method for many years and never had respiratory depression occurring in patients thus treated. Indeed the improvement in pain-free respiratory excursion and coughing have led to improved respiratory function, not worse. This regimen is different from most used in non-cardiothoracic patients but could well be adopted for these people since atelectasis and bronchopneumonia, for example, are common after abdominal surgery.

The technique of intravenous analgesia is therefore simple in its concepts and practice. The major problems lie in altering the attitudes of those immediately attending the patient and in creating a system in which the technique can be practised. The surgeon therefore needs to alter the expectations of the nursing staff concerning postoperative pain and to convince them of the real benefits of adequate analgesia. This process takes time, patience and persistence, and tests the surgeon's ability as a leader. Often the system needs changing as well. There is a danger that nurse managers, in particular, may be slow to appreciate what their clinical colleagues mean and may place administrative obstacles in the way of nurses giving intravenous medication. Changing such entrenched managerial attitudes can be done but demands a lot of effort and time.

Other Methods of Analgesia

Although intravenous analgesia is the most commonly used method, there are equally effective ways of controlling pain after cardiothoracic operations which are not so widely used at the moment. Thoracic epidural analgesia can be performed in centres accustomed to the practice of epidural analgesia in general and in these places is very effective indeed. Similarly, some centres have reported the use of intrathecal morphine administered by lumbar puncture as a means of controlling pain after cardiac surgery. In the foreseeable future, however, most hospitals will rely on intravenous analgesia for cardiothoracic patients. Perhaps one of the major advantages to hospitals of having cardiothoracic surgery will be gained when all postoperative patients have adequate analgesia by a simple regimen, no matter what operation they might have had.

The need for intensive analgesia lasts a few days only in cardiothoracic patients. Severe pain occurring after several days usually means some complication has occurred in the wound. In the median sternotomy, there is usually bone movement or infection as the cause and both will be detectable by clinical examination. Lateral thoracic wounds have at least two muscle layers below the skin and infection and abscess formation are difficult to detect in the early stages.

Bone movement occurring in a median sternotomy in the absence of infection should be treated conservatively, provided no respiratory or coughing difficulty is produced. Such mobility, although painful, will rapidly reduce over a period of a few days and the wound will become comfortable. Other painful complications are dealt with in Chapter 3.

Summary

Pain control after cardiothoracic operations allows adequate respiration and improves tracheobronchial toilet. Since the pain threshold of every patient is unique, analgesics have to be given according to individual requirements. Intravenous narcotics given in small, frequent doses will achieve pain control before respiratory depression occurs. Epidural and intrathecal analgesia is effective in skilled hands.

Conclusion

No patient should be allowed discomfort after an operation. Pain is of no value at this point and gives rise to serious complications.

Persisting Controversies

- Place of intrathecal morphine after open-heart surgery.
- Usefulness of self medication.
- The extended role of the nurse in the administration of intravenous analgesics.

Further reading

Harcus, A.W., Smith, R.B. & Whittle, B.A. (1977) *Pain.* London: Churchill Livingstone.

Matthews, E.T. & Abrams, L.D. (1981) Use of intrathecal morphine in cardiac surgery (Abstract). *Thorax, 36,* 76.

Shuman, R.L. & Peters, R.M. (1976) Epidural anaesthesia following thoracotomy in patients with chronic, obstructive airway disease. *J. Thorac. Cardiovasc. Surg., 71,* 82.

2 Complications of Pulmonary Surgery

Under the broad heading of pulmonary surgery, two main groups of operations are found. The first group is operations performed on the lungs themselves which usually consist of removal of part or the whole of one lung. These operations are performed for many congenital and acquired lesions. In Europe and North America, most lung resections are for treatment of neoplasms but in other parts of the world resections for chronic infections such as tuberculosis are proportionally more common. The second group of operations are those performed on the pleura with the object of allowing better function in the underlying lung. The excision of empyemas is the most obvious example but this group also includes relatively minor procedures which drain air or fluid from the pleural cavity.

Complications of pulmonary surgery may be caused either during investigation or during treatment.

Complications of Pulmonary Surgical Investigations

Bronchoscopy

The modern fibre-optic flexible bronchoscope is widely used under topical anaesthesia by physicians and has proved to be an extremely useful tool in the diagnosis of pulmonary disorders. The rigid metallic bronchosope, however, has not been made obsolete by the flexible instrument. The surgeon needs to know more than a diagnosis in lung disease and needs to know what is the best operation for that particular patient. This question can often only be settled by an assessment of the degree of rigidity in the bronchial tree around the lesion and clearly this information can only be obtained by using a rigid metallic bronchoscope.

Passage of the rigid bronchoscope into the respiratory tract is difficult unless the patient is completely relaxed. For most patients this means a general anaesthetic must be given but there are some phlegmatic individuals who can tolerate the procedure under topical anaesthesia only.

The anaesthetic is the first hazard. In order to relax the patient fully, neuromuscular blocking agents are used which stop spontaneous respirations. Clearly, there is danger in having a paralysed patient with a metallic viewing instrument in the airway. Danger also occurs because the investigation usually takes place in a darkened room where the anaesthetist may be impeded in early recognition of severe hypoxia, and cardiac arrest may occur.

Various ways have been used to oxygenate the patient and remove carbon dioxide during bronchoscopy under general anaesthetic. The most commonly used method now works on the Venturi principle (see Fig. 2.1). Oxygen is blown, under high pressure, through the narrow jet at the operator's end of the bronchoscope. The effect of this jet is to entrain air and the enhanced gas volume passes into the lungs and inflates them. The entrained air enters via the operator's viewing port and neither this nor the very narrow jet tube interfere with the operator's vision. Thus the examination may proceed with the surgeon getting a good view and with the patient adequately oxygenated. This technique has superseded methods such as intermittently inflating the lungs by an endotracheal tube jammed for a few seconds in the open end of the bronchoscope. However, even with the Venturi device, oxygenation may be abnormal and hypoxia may lead to a cardiac arrest. Consequently, bronchoscopy under general anaesthetic should be regarded as a major procedure and the possibility of cardiac arrest anticipated.

Passage of the bronchoscope

Soft tissue damage may be caused by the passage of the rigid, straight bronchoscope through the curves of the upper respiratory tract. This is undesirable in itself but later swelling of the pharynx, uvula or larynx may occur and cause upper respiratory obstruction. A non-traumatic passage of the bronchoscope can be performed by understanding the anatomy of the upper respiratory tract. The mouth lies at an angle of 110° to the pharynx and the larynx lies to the front of the hypopharynx. Thus passage of the rigid, straight bronchoscope means considerably increasing this angle (Fig. 2.1) and the combined manoeuvre is termed 'sniffing the morning air'. The angle between the mouth and the pharynx can be greatly increased by extension of the atlanto-occipital joint (see Fig. 2.1). This is achieved by firm traction on the patient's upper jaw by the gloved fingers of the surgeon's left hand. The bronchoscope is introduced beak forward with the surgeon's right hand (Fig. 2.2).

As the pharynx is entered, the bronchoscope tip is levered forwards using the surgeon's fingers as the fulcrum. The epiglottis is pushed anteriorly and the vocal cords seen. In order to pass the bronchoscope through them, it is rotated through 90° so that the beak lies towards the patient's right side. The trachea is then entered smoothly.

A frequent mistake when levering forward the soft tissues of the anterior wall of the pharynx is to allow the patient's teeth or alveolar margin to be the fulcrum rather than protecting them with the surgeon's fingers. Too much force is unnecessary; the thumb and two fingers of the right hand are sufficient to introduce the instrument.

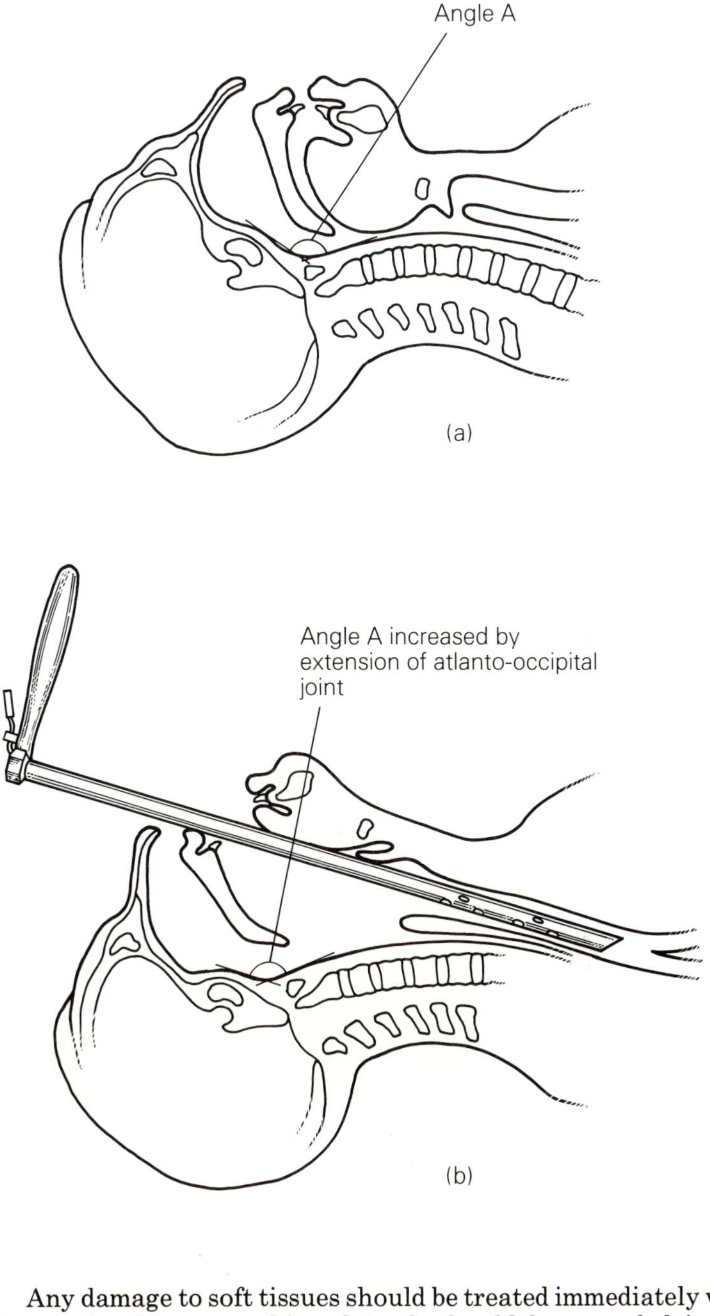

Figure 2.1
(a) Normal anatomy of upper respiratory tract and (b) distortions produced by insertion of the rigid bronchoscope. Note cervical lordosis, which is reduced by flexion, and angle A, which is increased by extension of the atlanto-occipital joint.

Any damage to soft tissues should be treated immediately with ice packs. Loose or chipped teeth should be recorded in the operative note. Throughout the operation, the surgeon's fingers should protect the upper teeth and alveolar margin.

Once the bronchoscope lies in the trachea, ventilation may commence and the major hazards of the procedure are passed.

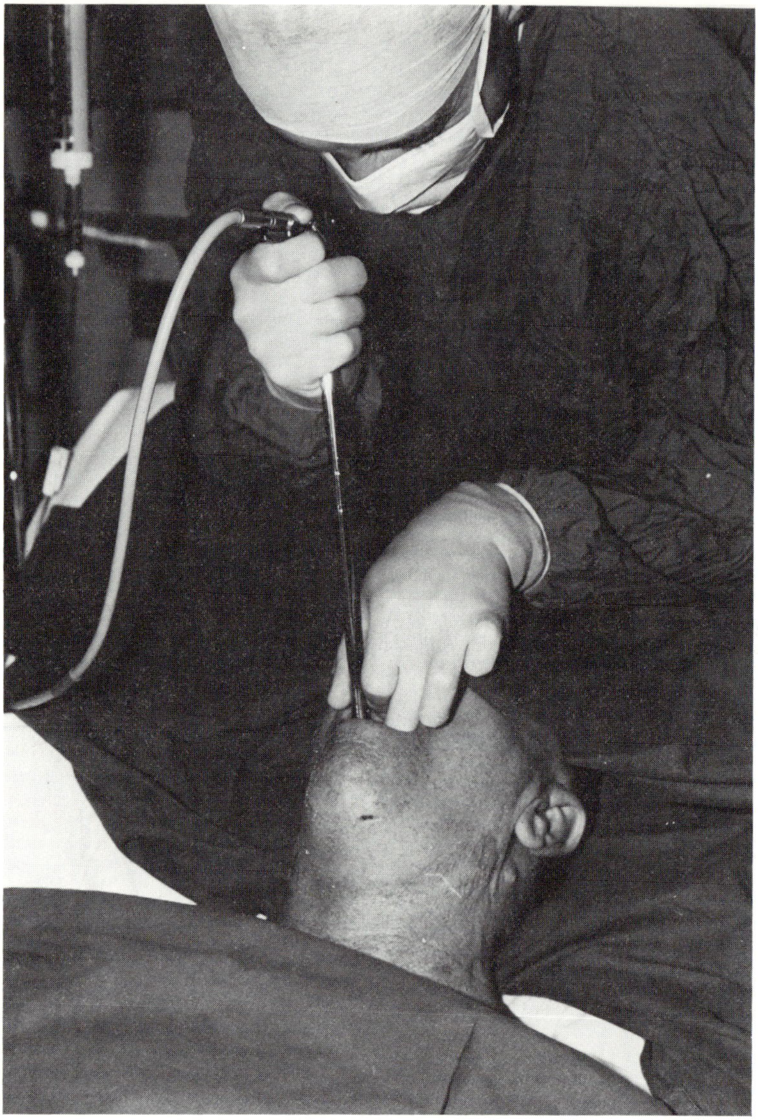

Figure 2.2
Introduction of the rigid bronchoscope under anaesthesia. Note the fingers of the left hand protecting the upper alveolar margin or teeth.

Bleeding If the bronchoscopy involves a bronchial biopsy, bleeding may be caused. This is dangerous not only because of blood loss but also because of the possiblity of shed blood flooding the bronchial tree and preventing oxygenation.

Certain points in the bronchial tree are very closely related to the pulmonary artery and its major branches, and biopsy at these points is therefore undertaken very carefully (Fig. 2.3). Given a choice, the prudent surgeon will try to biopsy as far posteriorly as possible and *always* under direct vision to avoid too large and too deep a bite with the biopsy forceps.

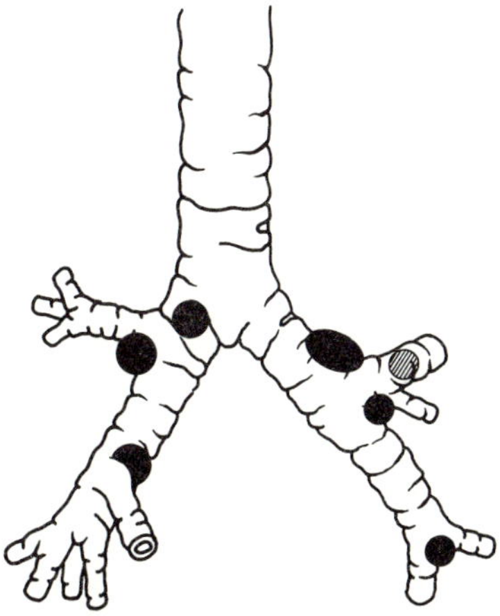

Figure 2.3
Areas of the bronchial tree which are very closely related to major pulmonary vessels and at which bronchial biopsy should be performed with extreme caution.

Should bleeding occur, the first priority is to prevent flooding of the remaining tree. A large efficient sucker is essential on the bronchoscopy tray for this reason. If after a five-minute period bleeding has not largely stopped, it is likely that a thoracotomy will have to be performed. While preparations for this are being made, a long endotracheal tube passed into the main bronchus on the side of the bleeding will at least prevent flooding of the other lung.

Lesser cases where the bleeding mostly stops should be allowed to breathe and cough, and nursed with the affected side downwards – the object again being to reduce flooding of the opposite lung.

Bronchography

This investigation allows the surgeon to assess the calibre and disease of the bronchial tree by the instillation of radiopaque medium into the bronchial tree. Any untoward reaction to the medium will cause swelling of the bronchial and tracheal mucosa, and this may lead to severe respiratory distress. Bronchography is a procedure to be performed with great caution.

First, the patient should be questioned about sensitivities, particularly to iodine compounds. Any positive history may have to be confirmed by a skin test and, if that is positive, another medium chosen. Second, physiotherapy should be given before and after the investigation in order to remove the medium rapidly from the bronchial tree. Finally, although bilateral bronchograms are permissible in adults, children should have one side at a time studied. The smaller size of the bronchial tree in children makes the margin of safety much smaller.

Mediastinoscopy

The purpose of mediastinoscopy is to identify and remove lymph nodes from the upper anterior mediastinum. The procedure is most commonly done as part of the assessment of the patient who has malignancy in the lung in order to assess the degree of spread to the mediastinum.

The procedure is performed under general anaesthesia through a small transverse incision 3 cm above the upper end of the sternum. The incision is carried down as far as the pretracheal fascia which is divided, allowing the finger or the endoscope into the thorax in the pretracheal plane. By blunt dissection, lymph nodes lying on the trachea as far down as the right main bronchus may be fully or partly removed.

Mediastinoscopy may lead to a failure to remove affected lymph tissue. Often the limitations of the procedure are not recognized. Lymph nodes to the left of the trachea are inaccessible and the procedure should only be performed if the answer lies in those nodes lying anteriorly or to the right of the trachea.

Bleeding is another potential problem. This may result from a biopsy of one of the major vascular structures in this part of the mediastinum such as the ascending aorta or innominate artery. Venous congestion, as in superior vena caval obstruction, will cause problems and mediastinoscopy should be avoided in patients with this syndrome. Some bleeding occurs in all patients having mediastinoscopy but usually ceases after a few minutes' pressure. Prolonged bleeding, especially if arterial, may require an emergency thoracotomy to locate its site and to stop the haemorrhage. If the haemorrhage is venous in origin, tilting the patient head-up will rapidly reduce it but care should be taken to prevent air embolism by closing or packing the wound first.

Thoracoscopy

Direct vision into the pleural cavity may allow diagnosis by recognition of lesions or by biopsy of such lesions. Thoracoscopy offers a small number of patients distinct benefits but is very infrequently performed nowadays. In order to introduce the thoracoscope into the pleural cavity it is necessary to introduce air into the pleural cavity to allow the lung to retract partially. Widespread pleural disease with obliteration of the space is therefore unsuitable for this procedure. Arterial air embolism is a remote but real possiblity when introducing air into the pleural cavity for any reason. It is probably caused by gas being forced into the pulmonary circulation, perhaps through a laceration of the lung which may not be visible or through a congenital weakness of the visceral pleura overlying the lung. The resultant embolism, passed through the circulation into the left side of the heart and thus into the arterial circulation, usually causes cerebral damage, the nature and severity of which is determined by the volume of air and chance, according to which part of the brain is embolized. Air embolism may be avoided by slowly introducing air into the pleural cavity and making sure that the instrument introducing the air is not in contact with or penetrating the lung.

Lung and bronchial biopsy

Every surgeon performing pulmonary surgery would prefer to operate on patients who have precise tissue diagnosis before the operation. This knowledge is necessary to plan the operation and to avoid needless risk. Thoracotomy performed without a precise diagnosis being made beforehand is always more hazardous than in other circumstances and may lead to unnecessary resections and loss of recoverable tissue. Ultimately, some patients will be judged to be more at risk from further investigations than from surgery, and operations will be performed, but these situations should be avoided if at all possible. Operating on a patient without a surgical lesion must be counted as a major and avoidable surgical complication.

Reference has already been made to bronchial biopsy performed through the bronchoscope and most lung neoplasms will continue to be diagnosed by this technique. Another reliable way of obtaining cells is by examination of a genuine specimen of sputum produced by the patient. Often a physiotherapist is needed to make sure that the specimen is sputum and not just saliva.

Approximately 20% of lung lesions lie beyond the reach of the flexible bronchoscope, lying peripherally in the lung. Percutaneous needle biopsy is frequently performed in order to get a tissue diagnosis and this, although extremely accurate and reliable, carries hazards.

The lesion is needled by a tissue biopsy needle introduced through the chest wall under biplane X-ray screening. Radiologists, therefore, frequently perform the investigation. After removal of the needle, pneumothorax may occur and is prone to develop tension complications. The suspicion of a pneumothorax being present should be high and further chest X-rays are indicated if any deterioration of the clinical situation occurs. A chest drain insertion set should always be available in the X-ray department and in the ward afterwards. About one-fifth of patients having a percutaneous lung biopsy will develop a pneumothorax and about one-half of these will need a drainage tube inserted for about 24 hours.

The complication of pneumothorax in lung biopsy is unavoidable but the early recognition and treatment of this complication will prevent damage to the patient.

Summary

Bronchoscopy, bronchography, mediastinoscopy, and lung and pleural biopsy yield a positive diagnosis in most cases of lung disease. Each has specific complications which are potentially life threatening. Full facilities for thoracotomy and chest drainage should be available, and the investigations should only be performed in an active thoracic surgical centre.

Conclusion
Every reasonable attempt must be made to establish a diagnosis before thoracotomy for lung disease. To remove too much lung tissue or to remove a lesion better treated medically is a major surgical complication.

Persisting controversies
- The role of 'blind' transbronchial lung biopsy.
- The indications for mediastinoscopy.
- Balancing the risks versus the benfits of preoperative investigation.

Complications of the Surgical Treatment of Lung Disease

Lesions in the lung needing an operation are usually excised with a greater or lesser amount of surrounding lung tissue. At one extreme a benign hamartoma may be shelled out of the lung, and at the other the whole lung may be removed.

Apart from the complications attending any major surgical procedure, such as pulmonary embolism, specific complications of lung surgery may arise from two sources. The direct complications of lung resection are considered here, and later (page 31) the complications of the thoracotomy operation itself will be considered.

Complications of lung resection
The majority of complications arising directly as a result of lung resection will be caused either by respiratory insufficiency or by bronchopleural fistula.

Respiratory insufficiency

Two factors may lead to inadequate lung function after pulmonary resection. First, there is loss of lung tissue which may lead to the patient having inadequate respiratory tissue remaining to support life or physical activity, even if all that tissue works normally. This is clearly a permanent situation and treatable only by avoiding it. Second, temporary loss of function may occur after surgery, however, and this is caused by handling the lung, by infection, by contusion and by the effects of transfused fluids. Given time, and if the patient survives, recovery will occur.

In respiratory failure occurring after lung surgery, a mixture of permanent and temporary factors is present. Clearly, the level of respiratory function before operation will determine if respiratory failure is likely to occur afterwards, and the decisions taken on this assessment will be crucial to the patient's survival.

Assessment of preoperative respiratory function. The aim is to estimate the severity of chronic generalized lung disease such as chronic bronchitis. The severity of dyspnoea should be carefully assessed when taking the history. Shortness of breath at rest or on mild exercise indicates poor respiratory reserve. Care must be taken to avoid patients minimizing this symptom. Since many have been dyspnoeic for so long, they fail to recognize normality. The duration of dyspnoea should be noted since some lung lesions needing surgery, such as collapse of a lobe or whole lung, will in themselves cause dyspnoea and yet be removable without the dyspnoea worsening. Such a situation is suggested by a short history of perhaps a few weeks. Similarly, clinical examination and the chest X-ray may suggest that dyspnoea may be due to the lesion itself and not to chronic generalized lung disease. An isolated 'lump' in the lung is unlikely to cause dyspnoea whereas a major area of atelectasis is at least a significant, if not the only, contribution to dyspnoea.

Laboratory tests of lung function need interpreting in the light of the clinical and radiological features. Detailed descriptions of the significance of abnormalities in lung volume, compliance and ventilation are available in other texts, as are the details of the measurement of gas transfer and lung perfusion. Some surgeons pay much attention to these tests, most very little. The adult patient with a forced vital capacity (FVC) of less than 2 l is unlikely to survive a thoracotomy and a peak expiratory flow rate (PEFR) of less than 200 l/min is worrying. Perhaps the major benefit of lung function studies is to identify the patient with a reversible airways obstruction.

The final decision on a patient's respiratory function takes into account all these different factors. The most important test is to observe and talk to a patient walking quickly over a fairly long distance – say 500–600 metres. The ability to carry on a conversation during this exercise usually means good respiratory function. The least useful tests are analysis of the arterial blood gases and ventilation–perfusion scans of the lung.

A further note of caution must be sounded. The assumption is that the contribution of the unaffected lung toward respiratory function is equal throughout. This may be wrong – and most of an 'adequate' respiratory function may reside in one part of the lungs and that may be the part about to be removed. Differential tests of the function in various lobes may be made but are cumbersome and not often done. The ultimate differential test is made at operation when the lung which is about to undergo surgery is collapsed. Respiratory insufficiency occurring at this stage should lead to the operation being abandoned.

Factors leading to temporary respiratory insufficiency. Handling, retraction and dissection of the surrounding healthy lung, as in a lobectomy, will cause considerable temporary lung damage and may cause respiratory failure.

Infection occurring in such lungs will have similar effects. Vigorous physiotherapy will prevent most infections, but commonly an antibiotic is given as well – usually a broad spectrum type. Once infection does occur, vigorous antibiotic treatment is given along with physiotherapy and perhaps bronchoscopy to remove bronchial secretions. The importance of a strong pain-free cough in clearing bronchial secretions and avoiding collapse and infection must be recognized. Adequate pain control and good physiotherapy will minimize any tendency towards pulmonary infection.

Fluid administration during and after surgery may damage the lungs in two ways. First, excessive volumes of crystalloid solutions as favoured by some anaesthetists may lead to pulmonary interstitial oedema and 'stiff' lungs. Second, blood given may contain microemboli which end up in the microcirculation of the pulmonary bed. These two causes of respiratory dysfunction are avoidable. Large volumes of clear fluids should be avoided and all blood should be filtered through a microfilter, many types of which are commercially available.

Recognition of respiratory insufficiency after lung operation. Respiratory insufficiency after surgery is often missed and the patient subsequently has an 'unexplained' cardiac arrest or a 'stormy' postoperative course. The reasons for missing the diagnosis are to be found in the varying and subtle ways in which respiratory insufficiency may present.

Frank cyanosis is rare. Usually, the clinical picture is of a slowly deteriorating patient with a slowly rising respiratory rate. The patient may be confused or anxious. The pulse may become rapid for no accountable reason, or atrial fibrillation or flutter may be detected on the electrocardiogram. The blood pressure may suddenly increase. The cough and ability to co-operate with the physiotherapist become weaker. Detailed clinical examination of the chest leads to a similar variety of confusing and individually unimportant physical signs. Accumulation of secretions in the airways and an increasing area of bronchial breathing are common. The chest X-ray usually shows some increase in shadowing at both bases.

The important point to emphasize is that there is no one pathognomonic sign of respiratory failure. In its early stages, the number and variety of clinical signs is very confusing. The appearance of the patient from the bottom of the bed is very important. The attitude of the surgeon should be that any unexplained deviation from normal in the patient should be attributed to respiratory insufficiency in the first place, and only when this is ruled out should other causes or symptomatic treatment be considered.

The most reliable way of confirming respiratory insufficiency is to measure the tensions of oxygen and carbon dioxide in the patient's arterial blood. Oxygen levels of below 10 kPa and carbon dioxide levels of above 7 kPa together represent respiratory failure. Some patients will, by overbreathing, maintain a barely adequate oxygen tension of around 10 kPa, but the carbon dioxide tension will fall to below 4 kPa. This particular derangement of the blood gases is important because sudden deterioration may follow.

Most cardiothoracic surgical units have the means to measure arterial blood gases available either in the ward or nearby. An aggressive policy of measuring the blood gases in the early management of every unwell patient should be encouraged. Only then will early respiratory failure be detected. The most common reason for respiratory failure not to be detected is failure to consider the possibility and the next most common is a failure to measure the arterial blood gases.

Treatment of respiratory insufficiency. This should be performed as a combined treatment by the surgeon and the anaesthetist since, in the most severe cases, ventilator treatment may be needed. Indeed, the anaesthetist has the major contribution to make, but the surgeon should not abdicate his responsibilities entirely – the principles on which the treatment is based should at least be understood.

In early respiratory failure, effective treatment may consist merely of increasing the level of inspired oxygen by means of a face mask. Physiotherapy, pain control and the antibiotic treatment of infection are given where appropriate. Frequent clinical and blood gas assessments are made in order to assess the effectiveness of these treatments. The very tired patient with a weak cough will respond inadequately to physiotherapy, and bronchoscopic suction under topical anaesthesia may quickly remove retained bronchial secretions.

Just when such simple treatments must be abandoned and ventilator treatment commenced is a matter of judgement and varies from surgeon to surgeon. Surgical pride and worry about the adverse effects of ventilation on the postoperative patient often lead to delay in beginning artificial ventilation. There can be no doubt that increasing the intrathoracic pressure reduces cardiac output; similarly, bronchial suture lines may be disrupted by the procedure and the patient's discomfort will be increased by the insertion of an endotracheal tube for the purposes of ventilation. All these factors must be considered before starting artificial ventilation. To delay unduly, however, is to damage the patient, possibly irreversibly. The beneficial effects of ventilation are to remove the work of respiration from the exhausted patient and to reverse the effects of hypoxia and hypercapnia. In addition, the endotracheal tube offers a ready access for the removal by suction of bronchial secretions.

The decision to ventilate artificially is easy if simple measures fail to arrest progressive deterioration of the clinical situation or blood gases. The problem lies in the patient who is just about managing with simple treatments. Local factors such as the skill and numbers of nursing and medical staff then have to be considered. In most cases, ventilation is probably unduly delayed. However, to routinely ventilate patients with respiratory difficulties is obviously wrong. The best interests of the patient are served by the surgeon and anaesthetist agreeing on the time of ventilation.

Artificial ventilation should be carried out on an intensive care ward because of the numbers of nursing staff available and their special skills. Patients undergoing ventilation for respiration failure should have an indwelling arterial cannula inserted, usually into a radial artery at the wrist. This allows constant measurement of the arterial pressure and provides an access for repeated arterial blood samples. A central venous presure cannula is also needed. A nasogastric tube is inserted, thus allowing decompression of the stomach or, later on, enteral feeding. An urinary catheter is usually inserted to allow for easier nursing.

An endotracheal tube is usually inserted for ventilation purposes. The practice on our unit has been to insert this through the mouth, the nasal route having been abandoned because of pressure problems caused by the tube to the nostrils. Endotracheal intubation is uncomfortable and patients need a combination of analgesia and sedation. Omnopon is used on our unit and we give this by intravenous injection in small amounts (say 5 mg) as often as necessary. Patients who are hypoxic may need very large amounts initially. Some units use constant infusion techniques to administer drugs such as fentanyl with success. Only in extreme cases have we used muscle relaxants to paralyse the restless patient.

The endotracheal tube has an air cuff designed to prevent leakage. Over-distension of this will cause pressure necrosis of the trachea and subsequent stricture formation. Most units have a policy that the minimum amount of inflation possible is used and that adjustments to the amount are only made by a senior anaesthetist. We have used such a policy for 15 years and never had a problem with tracheal ulceration or stricture.

When respiratory failure needs ventilation, recovery usually takes some days before spontaneous respiration is effective. In severe cases this may take several weeks. In this period, problems arise relating to the general care of the patient and to the local respiratory condition.

Nutrition has to be maintained. As soon as the gut begins to recover from the ileus which is common in respiratory failure, enteral liquid feeding may begin via the nasogastric tube. Before that, however, parenteral feeding should be considered. Ventilated patients have a high nutritional requirement and this must be met by one means or another.

Absence of an effective cough and the presence of a foreign body in the trachea predisposes to pulmonary infection. A strict aseptic technique must be maintained in endotracheal suction and the sputum must be constantly examined by the bacteriologist. Some degree of contamination of the respiratory tract is inevitable, however, and the decision to start antibiotic treatment should only be made when infection occurs as shown by the systemic reaction of the patient. Too early and too broad an antibiotic will lead to proliferation of non-sensitive organisms such as *Pseudomonas aeruginosa* and other Gram-negative bacteria.

The physiotherapist is vital during periods of prolonged ventilation. A combination of postural drainage and forcible expulsion of secretions by percussion and vibration is slowly effective in clearing the lungs and preventing accumulation of sputum.

If the patient is ventilated for a long time and is likely to need ventilation for a further period, tracheostomy should be considered. Although this involves surgical trauma to the trachea, once performed it allows greater patient comfort, easier nutrition and the ability to reduce or withdraw narcotics. Our policy has been to perform tracheostomy if ventilation is likely to continue for more than one week, but many other policies are found in other units which are equally effective.

As the condition of the patient improves, spontaneous ventilation must be allowed. Usually, short periods are permitted to become longer until eventually the patient is extubated. If the ventilation has been performed for a long time, the patient will need a prolonged period of weaning to build up his respiratory muscles again and the process of becoming completely independent of ventilation may take several weeks. At the other extreme, a patient with a very short period of ventilation and an easily remedied cause of respiratory failure may be extubated within minutes of ceasing to be ventilated. After extubation, vigorous efforts are needed in order to prevent respiratory failure recurring and a period of several days of intensive nursing and physiotherapy is needed.

Summary

Respiratory insufficiency is common after lung surgery and is due to a combination of permanent and temporary drainage. Before operation, every effort should be made to identify those patients with chronic lung disorders who will be unable to tolerate further loss of lung function. A combination of clinical and laboratory criteria are used, but the ultimate test is the ability of the patient to survive on one lung during surgery.

After operation, temporary exacerbation of respiratory insufficiency may occur and adequate pain control, physiotherapy and oxygen are essential. The diagnosis of respiratory failure is often very difficult and no single pathognomonic test is available. Ventilator treatment may be needed to allow treatment of those factors causing temporary pulmonary dysfunction.

Conclusion

Before operation, a detailed assessment will help to avoid

operation on those patients with inadequate respiratory function. After operation, vigorous treatment of the lungs is needed to reduce the effect of temporary factors, further diminishing lung function. The diagnosis of respiratory failure is often unduly delayed and leads to considerable mortality and morbidity.

Persisting controversies

- The usefulness of laboratory tests of respiratory function.
- The value of the exercise test.
- The role of blood gas analysis in the early detection of respiratory failure.
- The timing and frequency of bronchoscopic removal of secretions.
- The timing of tracheostomy.

Bronchopleural fistula

Any communication between the bronchial air space and the pleural cavity is a bronchopleural fistula. The term is usually reserved, however, for those communications which occur following repair of the bronchus after removal of a lobe or the whole lung, i.e. those arising as a complication of pulmonary resection.

The main bronchus and its major segmental branches receive their blood supply from the bronchial arteries which arise directly from the descending aorta. Two or three major bronchial arteries pass in the peribronchial tissues of the main bronchus and branch into the major segmental peribronchial tissues. Each gives off small branches which supply the adjacent bronchus, but there is a poor network of vessels within the bronchial wall. The net result is a rather poorly vascularized tissue, which is similar in healing powers and its susceptibility to avascular necrosis as the colon. Surgical trauma to the bronchus, which occurs as a result of incision and surgical repair, therefore often leads to areas of avascular necrosis and consequent disruption of the suture line.

Bacterial contamination of the bronchial tree is normally present from the larynx down to bronchiolar level. Thus any ischaemic or avascular areas readily become infected and when the bronchial repair disrupts, infection will spread to the pleural cavity. After a pneumonectomy, the thorax is empty on the affected side and the infection rapidly becomes permanently established. Thus a bronchopleural fistula after pneumonectomy causes problems due to infection and due to air leakage from the bronchial tree. Postlobectomy bronchopleural fistulas are less serious since the pleural cavity is occupied by the expanded remaining lung and theoretically, at least, no space remains. Thus infection is more readily controlled by the body's natural defences and the only remaining problem is one of air leak.

Prevention of bronchopleural fistula. The tendency of the surgically repaired bronchus to disrupt is influenced by a number of factors, the most important of which is surgical technique. The blood supply to the bronchus is not rich and individual variability may make it even more sparse, thus increasing the tendency to form a fistula. However, a surgical technique which recognizes this, and at all stages treates the bronchus appropriately, will lead to a very low incidence of bronchopleural fistula.

The underlying purpose of any technique must be to preserve the blood supply to the bronchus. No mechanical clamps must be placed on the bronchus which is to be left in the patient, although it is permissible to apply a bronchial clamp distally on the bronchus which can be removed in order to prevent spillage of secretions. A precise dissection of the bronchus will strip peribronchial tissue containing bronchial arteries. It is much more desirable to avoid a precise dissection and identify the bronchus by touch. Using a sharp knife, the bronchus and the peribronchial tissues are cut cleanly across. There is usually some bleeding, and the vessels are identified and ligated individually. Diathermy is unreliable on these vessels and again may damage other tissue.

Suture repair of the bronchus is then performed. Material which does not cause any inflammation, and consequently the need for increased blood supply, is used. Most units use stainless steel wire. Interrupted simple sutures are used and placed in such a manner that closure is achieved with minimal disturbance to the blood supply (Fig. 2.4). The ideal suture is unabsorbable and either made of stainless steel or any monofilament synthetic suture. Each stitch encompasses a perfect cube of tissue. In this way, closure may be achieved without creating ischaemia. Many units use the automatic stapler to close bronchial stumps and

Figure 2.4
One method of suturing the bronchial stump by hand.

x = Thickness of tissue
= Depth of stitch
= Distance between stitches

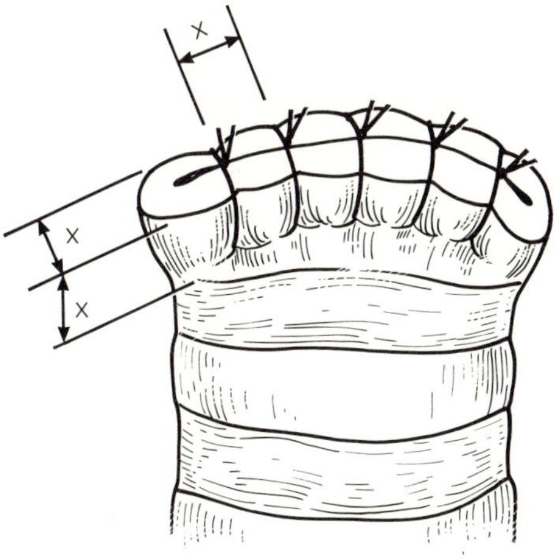

Figure 2.5
Chest X-rays showing the occurrence of a large bronchopleural fistula after left pneumonectomy. The patient coughed up 1500 ml of brown fluid and became acutely ill in the interval between film (a) and film (b) (opposite). At operation, a large fistula was closed.

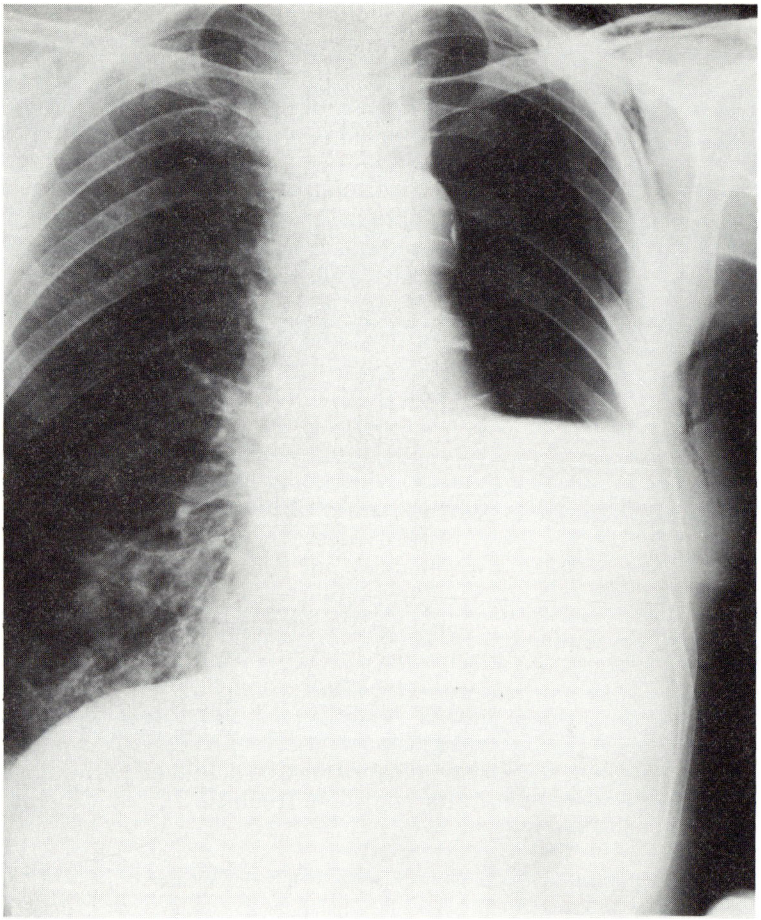

(a)

there is some published evidence that the incidence of fistulas is reduced. This has not been the experience of other units and we rely on manual suture techniques.

After the repair is completed, its closure is confirmed by submerging the suture line under clear fluid and asking the anaesthetist to inflate the remaining lung via the endotracheal tube. Pressures of up to 60 mmHg (8.0 kPa) should be used. Any residual air leak should be closed by further interrupted simple stainless steel wire sutures.

Following repair, the postpneumonectomy stump is buried under tissue. We have used a pedicle graft of the intercostal muscle, but others use a flap of pleura. Several stitches bury the bronchus stump under the non-bronchial tissue and thereby should help to discourage fistula formation. However, evidence as to this latter point is lacking. Similarly, powdered antibiotics applied around the repaired bronchus are widely used but of no proven help.

Figure 2.5 (b)

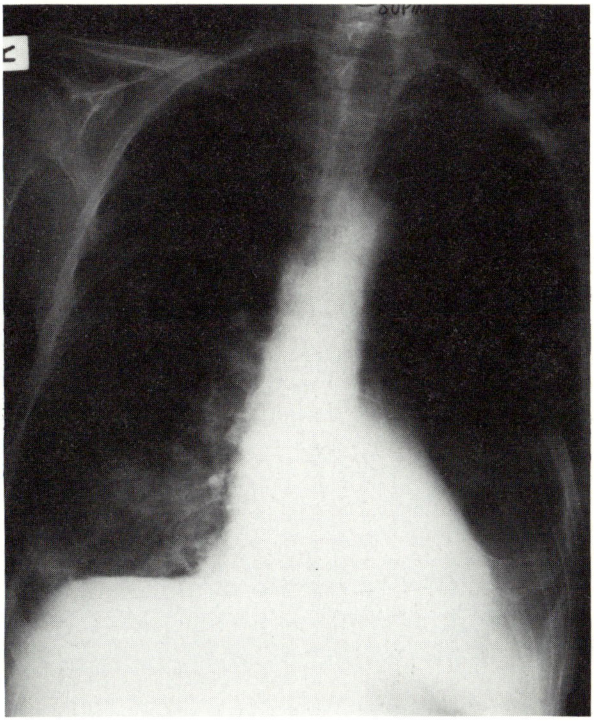

Diagnosis of postpneumonectomy bronchopleural fistula. If the bronchial suture line develops a large defect, the diagnosis of the fistula is easy. Suddenly, at 8–12 days after surgery, the patient coughs up a large volume of dark brown liquid. Often some of this will spill over into the opposite remaining lung and cause severe respiratory distress. A chest X-ray will show that the level of fluid in the hemithorax has fallen dramatically (Fig. 2.5). There are few more straightforward situations in thoracic surgery. Should the fistula be a small one, however (perhaps no more than 1 or 2 mm in diameter), diagnosis becomes extremely difficult.

The volume of space fluid lost through a small fistula is very low and may never be coughed up. Instead it passes into the remaining lung, and by causing inflammation is absorbed. The inflammatory process in the opposite lung usually affects the lower lobe and may be treated as pneumonia. Similarly, the volume of fluid lost through a small fistula may be less than the volume being secreted into the empty hemithorax; thus the level of fluid in the hemithorax may not decrease as expected, therefore adding to diagnostic difficulties.

The real clue to diagnosis lies in the air space above the fluid in the hemithorax on the operated side. Normally after a pneumonectomy, this air space is progressively smaller and always under negative pressure. Clinically and radiologically, the mediastinum is deviated towards that side and on X-ray the space

Figure 2.6
(a) Chest X-ray taken on ninth day after right peumonectomy. Note shape of air space – triangular shape indicates negative pressure.
(b) Chest X-ray of the same patient one day later. Note altered shape of air space indicating positive pressure. Fluid level has not significantly fallen. At operation, a small bronchopleural fistula was found.

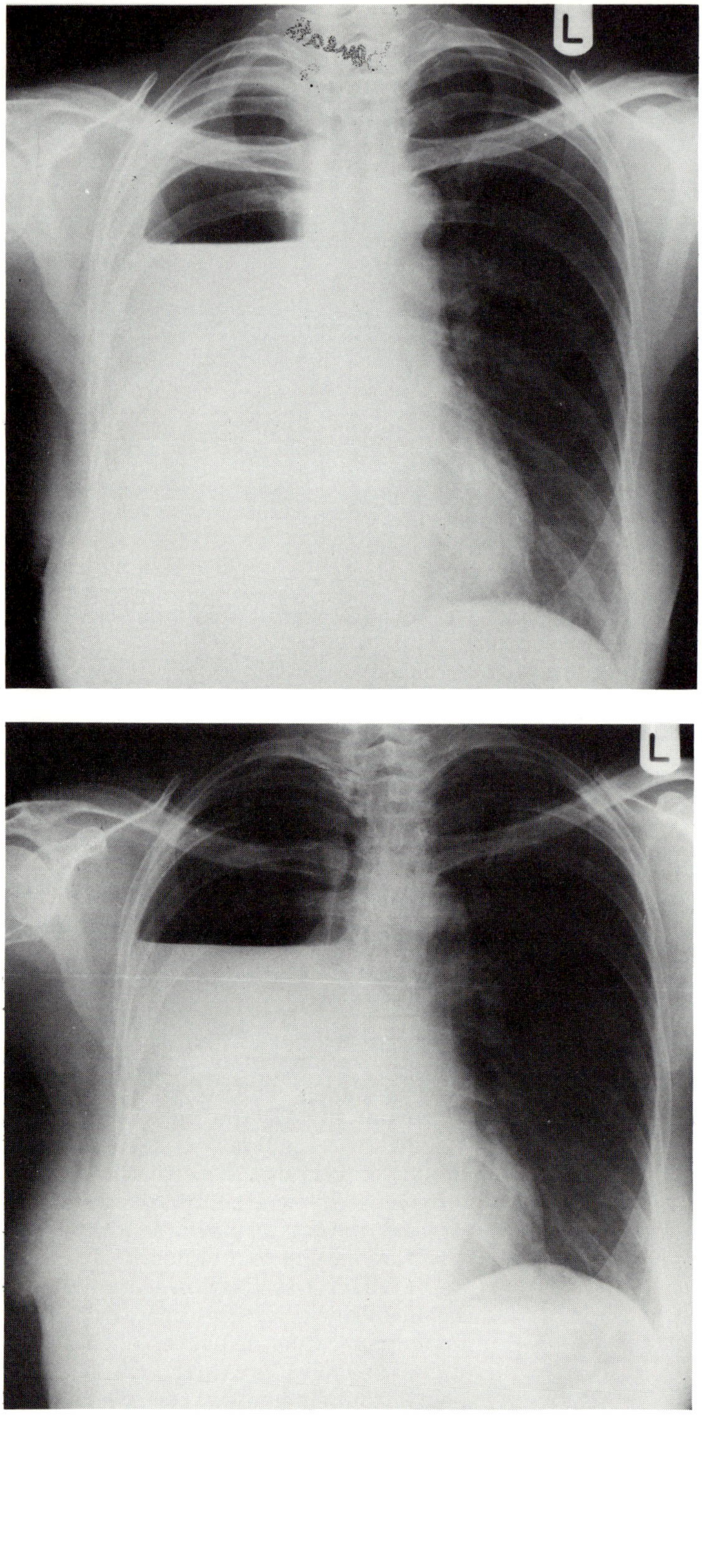

(a)

(b)

has a characteristic triangular shape. If a small fistula is present, air leaks in from the trachea, the pressure increases causing the mediastinum to revert to the midline, and the shape of the air space on the chest X-ray becomes almost semicircular. Clearly, such subtle radiological signs may only be appreciated by close comparison of comparable films taken at intervals (Fig. 2.6).

The diagnosis of the 'small' bronchopleural fistula is important because the fistula will cause prolonged severe morbidity. The inflammatory process in the remaining lung may become infected. The pneumonectomy space itself will become infected, leading to a postpneumonectomy empyema – one of the most difficult problems of thoracic surgery. Early repair of the fistula is indicated when the radiological signs above are found. The repair is achieved by excision of the whole suture line and resuturing of fresh bronchial stump.

The practice of injecting methylene blue or another dye into the pneumonectomy space in order to detect a bronchopleural fistula is misleading at best. The fluid in a pneumonectomy space rapidly becomes loculated by fibrin partitions and injected methylene blue may well not be found in the sputum, even if the bronchopleural fistula is a large one.

Other bronchopleural fistulas occurring after lung resection. The underlying cause of the fistula remains the same as that of postpneumonectomy lesions. The major and beneficial difference lies in the fact that after lobectomy, segmentectomy or wedge resection, there is the remaining lung on the operated side which expands after surgery to fill the cavity of the hemithorax. General surgical principles, therefore, suggest that the inevitable contamination by bacteria passing through the fistula into the hemithorax will cause infection only with great difficulty – *provided the lung is fully expanded.* The problem of the air leak of course remains, but as long as a drainage tube allows this to be removed, and the lung stays fully expanded, ultimately the fistula will heal. Operation only becomes necessary when the volume of air leaking through the fistula is so great as to prevent full expansion of the remaining lung. The use of the stapler when removing portions of lung will avoid many small bronchopleural fistulas.

Summary of treatment of bronchopleural fistulas

1 *Large postpneumonectomy fistula:*

(a) Lie the patient on the affected side.
(b) Insert a chest drain to remove remaining fluid.
(c) Give general support – antibiotics, oxygen, nutrition.
When the condition of the patient improves, either:
(d) Operative repair of the fistula if there is little contamination of the pleural space, or

(e) Fenestration of the chest wall, involving removal of segments of at least 3 cm to permit dependent drainage.

Local antiseptic washouts are then used until the infection is controlled and all slough has discharged. At this time, which may be months afterwards, the fistula may be closed and the chest wall repaired. Filling the empty hemithorax with 0.25% neomycin solution in saline has been used with success.

2 *Small postpneumonectomy fistula.* Treat as for large fistula, but with an emphasis on early repair.

3 *Fistula occurring after other lung resections:*

(a) Drain the pleural cavity with large underwater seal drains and apply suction to encourage lung expansion.

(b) If the chest X-ray shows full expansion and no empty space in hemithorax, maintain suction until the pleural layers are fused – about 20 days.

(c) Stop suction. If the lung remains fully expanded, cut the drain short and let it discharge into a dressing pack strapped to the chest wall.

(d) With X-ray control, withdraw the tube slowly – maximum rate 5 cm every two weeks.

Conclusion

Bronchopleural fistula after lung resection is due to poor healing of the divided bronchus. The nature of its blood supply leads to the bronchus being highly susceptible to surgical trauma. Appropriate techniques will reduce the incidence of the complication. Postpneumonectomy bronchopleural fistula is extremely difficult to treat because of the empty hemithorax and because the complication usually follows a resection for bronchial neoplasm. Early fistulas are repaired immediately, but those occurring late may need expectant treatment until the course of the underlying neoplasm is determined.

Persisting controversies

- The role of the chest X-ray in diagnosing small fistulas.
- The ideal method of bronchial repair.
- The type of treatment needed in the management of the late bronchopleural fistula.

Postoperative chest drainage

Drainage of the chest cavity after pulmonary surgery is the major cause of worry to the junior staff and those beginning in the specialty. The procedure is thought to be uniquely complicated and each individual tends to have different ideas of the objectives of such procedures. Although chest drainage is not strictly a complication of pulmonary surgery, complications will inevitably arise if the management of the drains is faulty because of poor understanding. Furthermore, the principles of postoperative chest drainage apply to any form of chest drainage for other conditions and will be considered here.

The lungs are elastic and left to themselves contract into small airless balls of tissue. Full expansion in the intact human is achieved by the fact that the pleural 'cavity' is non-existent; this is because the visceral and parietal pleura remain in contact with each other and offer great resistance to separation by virtue of a pressure which is below atmospheric (−5 mmHg). Clearly, any tendency of the lung to retract from the chest wall greatly increases the negative pressure thus maintaining full expansion. The full expansion of the lung thus depends on an intact lung, an intact chest wall and a pleural space which is potential rather than actual.

The purpose of postoperative pleural drainage is to maintain the pleural cavity as potential in spite of breaches in the lung and chest wall and the possibility of accumulation of fluids and air in the pleural cavity (Fig. 2.7). Thus the drains in the chest after surgery have to be designed to allow air, blood and fluid to flow freely out of the chest and yet prevent the entry of air into the low-pressure pleural cavity. Failure to achieve this will lead to collapse of the underlying lung and its loss of function. Equally important, the positive pressure in one hemithorax will push the mediastinum to the opposite good lung, further impairing respiratory function. Thus inadequate pleural drainage after surgery

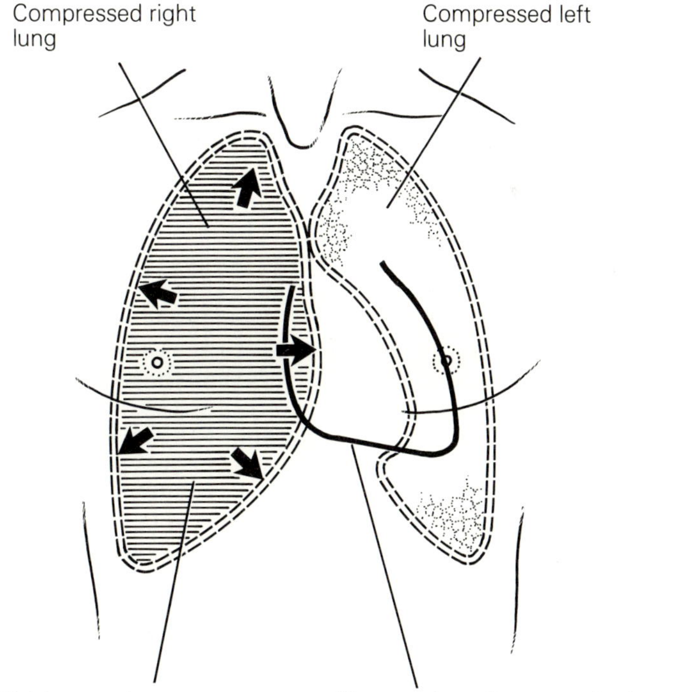

Figure 2.7 Effects of fluid or gas under tension in the pleural cavity. Shift of the mediastinum causing compression of the opposite lung interferes with ventilation and the term 'tension' is applied to this condition. Kinking of the major vessels is unlikely to cause the severity of problems which follow.

will lead to problems in both lungs, operated and 'healthy' (see Fig. 2.7).

The drains are tubular and are pulled through the chest wall at the time of surgery. If only blood is expected to drain, a drainage tube lying just above the diaphragm is sufficient. If air leakage is anticipated, a second drainage tube is inserted through a separate incision and adjusted so that its end lies high in the pleural cavity. If two drains are inserted, a known arrangement should be adopted to avoid confusing one with the other. The usual practice is to place the *A*nterior drain to the *A*pex in order to drain *A*ir, and the *B*asal drain is placed at the *B*ack to drain *B*lood.

Inert plastic materials or rubber can be used for drainage tubes. There is some advantage in rubber because it is slightly irritant and promotes pleural fusion. The open external end of the drain must be attached to a system which allows fluid and air to get out of the chest freely and yet which does not permit air to return into the chest (Fig. 2.8). This is achieved as shown in Fig. 2.8 by placing the tube under a water seal. By altering the amount of water in the bottle, the height of the negative pressure in the thorax can be determined.

There are various surgical opinions regarding the merits of suction applied to chest drains. Some believe that suction promotes and prolongs the leakage of air and blood. If the prime importance of achieving full lung expansion is appreciated, however, suction will be applied even if there is an increase in the drainage for a while. Our practice has been to apply suction to every postoperative chest drain. Low negative pressures (–5–10 mmHg) are applied to promote the drainage of fluids, but a higher negative pressure (–30 mmHg) is used if there is an air leak as well.

Usually chest drainage ceases after a few days and the drains are then removed – usually with the precaution of pre- and postoperative chest X-rays to ensure that the lung remains expanded. Sometimes the drainage continues, however, and consequently the drains are left in. About 15–20 days after surgery, the pleural cavity is obliterated by fibrous adhesions in most patients. At this time the chest drains may be cut short and allowed to drain into a dressing. The tendency of the lung to collapse will be prevented by pleural symphysis. The drains may then be slowly removed as in a non-thoracic surgical case.

Complications of chest drainage

1 *Insertion of chest drains at the bedside.* The insertion of a chest drain at the bedside is dangerous only if certain rules are not obeyed. These rules are:

(a) Drains are only inserted if a chest X-ray shows either a pneumothorax or haemothorax with separation of the visceral and parietal pleura.

(b) The drain must not be inserted too high, too low or too centrally. This is achieved by inserting the drain in the area

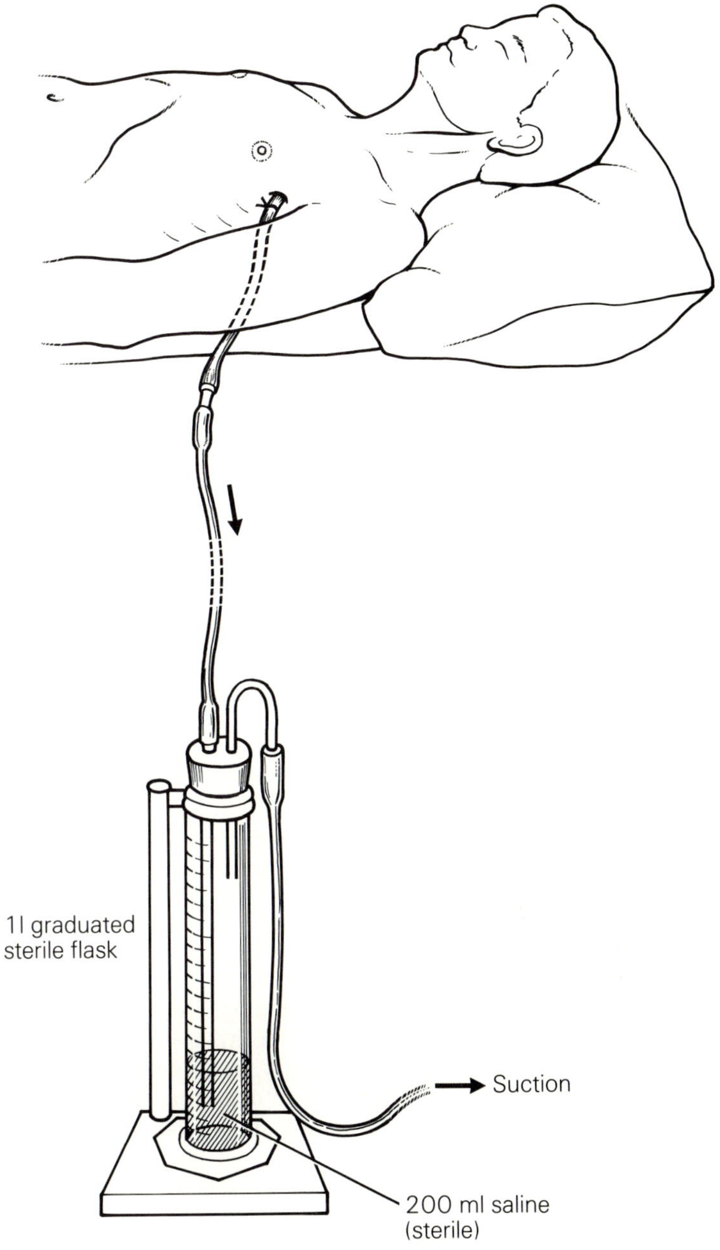

Figure 2.8 Principle of underwater seal closed-chest drainage. The site of insertion is shown in the 'triangle of safety' (see Fig. 2.9).

shown in the diagram (Fig. 2.9). In this position, there is very little danger of damage to intrathoracic or chest wall structure, the muscles are relatively thin and the position creates maximal patient comfort without any subsequent unsightly scar. Even if the diaphragm is elevated, it is unlikely to reach the lower limit of the area shown.

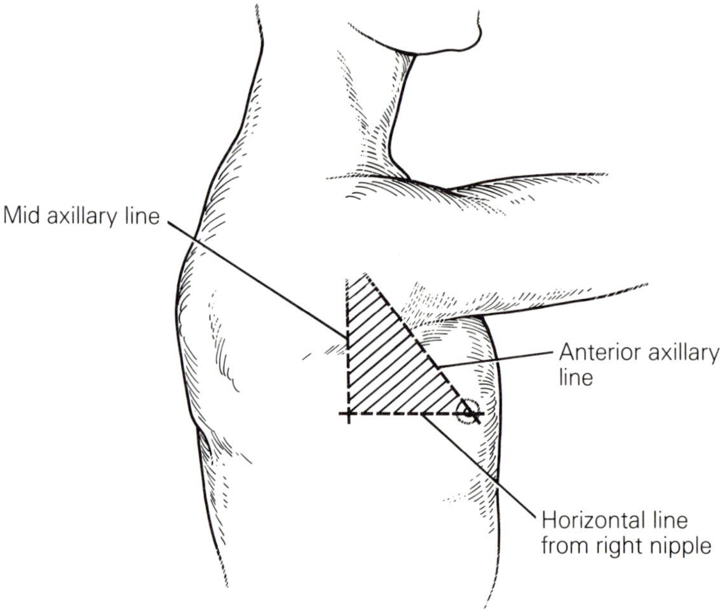

Figure 2.9
The 'triangle of safety'. This is the best site for insertion of needles or chest drains through the chest wall into the pleural cavity.

The practice of inserting chest drains into the anterior second left interspace should be abandoned. It is dangerous and uncomfortable for the patient, and overlies a bulky muscle mass and, potentially, an abnormally lateral internal mammary artery.

(c) Adequate anaesthesia of the chest wall should be achieved before the procedure is begun. The sensitivity of the parietal pleura should be remembered and at least 20 ml of 1% lignocaine is needed at least *five* minutes before the insertion begins.

2 *Failure of the drains to 'work'*. The objective of chest drainage must be remembered, i.e. to achieve full expansion of the underlying lung. If this fails to happen and the drain is lying in the pleural cavity, only two reasons can be present. Either fluid or air is accumulating at a rate greater than that at which it can be removed, *or* the underlying lung is incapable of expansion.

Most cases of failure of the drains to 'work' are caused by collapse of the underlying lung and not by inadequacy of the drainage system. The treatment, therefore, is to remove the cause of the collapse which usually means that bronchial obstruction must be treated by bronchoscopy. Manipulation of drains is rarely effective.

Clearly, chest drains will also fail to remove substances from the pleural cavity which are not fluid. Clotted blood is the most obvious example; this will often need a thoracotomy to remove it and allow full expansion of the lung. Expansion of the lung may be prevented by the solid fibrin slough which accompanies an empyema, and which is part of the localization process in the body's defences against spreading infection. Removal of the liquid pus by drainage fails to produce full expansion of the underlying lung and then only open surgical removal of the slough will achieve its removal. The earlier that pus is drained from the pleural cavity the less likely it is that slough will have formed. Thus the urgency of draining an empyema – usually on the day of diagnosis – is to avoid the necessity for a formal decortication operation.

Plan for the management of the 'failed' chest drain

Diagnosis by chest X-ray showing failure of the lung to expand

1 Check that the drain is lying in the pleural cavity, that it is connected correctly to the underwater seal and that suction is being applied.
2 If air or fluid is leaking rapidly from the chest for more than a short period after the drain is inserted, thoracotomy is indicated in order to control the source.
3 If no air or fluid is leaking through the drain, either collapse of the underlying lung (most likely) or solid material in the pleural cavity is present. Therefore perform bronchoscopy and remove retained bronchial secretions. If a further X-ray shows no improvement and collapse is still present, repeat bronchoscopy in six hours and start intensive physiotherapy. If a chest X-ray shows solid material in the pleural cavity it will need a thoracotomy at some time to remove it.
4 Only rarely should the failed chest drain be repositioned or replaced.

Faulty removal of chest drains

The technique or timing of chest drain removal may cause complications. A chest X-ray taken immediately before, and another taken immediately afterwards, are therefore essential.

Technique

The removal requires two people. The first person clamps the drain and cuts the retaining stitch holding the drain in position. The second person is needed to tie the longer second stitch, which has been placed at the time of insertion of the drain, so that the incision in the chest wall can be made airtight. As the chest drain is removed the patient is instructed to take a deep breath and hold it, thus raising the intrathoracic pressure above atmospheric. The drain is then smoothly pulled out of the chest by the first person and the stitch tied by the second. The patient is then asked to breathe normally.

Timing

In common with all other drains, chest drains are removed when they are no longer functioning (i.e. drainage has ceased).

If the chest drain has been inserted to drain fluid, the timing of the removal is easy. Once the drainage is down to about 10–20 ml/h, the tube should be removed. If the original problem was non-infective (as for instance in a haemothorax), the removal is completed very quickly in one operation.

Pus drainage tubes should be removed very slowly so that loculation does not occur. Removal of the empyema drainage tube should only begin when full expansion of the underlying lung is accomplished and demonstrated by a sinogram performed via the tube. Thereafter, the tube is removed by about 5 cm every two weeks, always provided that repeated sinograms are performed. Thus removal may take many weeks, but because of pleural fusion the tube may be shortened externally and allowed to drain into a soft dressing.

If the chest drainage tube was inserted in order to remove air, the timing of its removal is more difficult and depends on the nature of the original pneumothorax. In the younger patient with a spontaneous pneumothorax, the drain usually stops bubbling air when the lung expands. After a 24-hour period, the drain may then be removed as described above. Many older patients with pneumothorax have severe underlying lung disease such as emphysema. The diseased lung expands less readily and the air leak from it tends to stop only slowly. Thus removal of the tube may have to be delayed for some weeks. When the leak of air stops, it is wise to be very cautious about removing the drain quickly. A good plan is to clamp the drain for 24 or 48 hours after the last air bubble and then perform another X-ray in order to confirm that the underlying lung is still fully expanded. If so, the drain is removed. Frequently, however, a pneumothorax will be present and a further period of chest drainage required. This is accomplished by unclamping the drain.

In some patients, the air leak continues for many weeks. It is then a matter of surgical judgement whether a thoracotomy should be performed and the air leak closed or whether drainage should be continued until pleural symphysis occurs. This decision depends on the age and condition of the patient and the nature of the underlying lung disease. The risk of prolonged immobilization must be considered and the experience and skills of the operating surgeon. In the right hands thoracotomy will shorten the illness and is associated with less risk, but circumstances may indicate the non-operative approach. If a non-operative means is used, the drain should be connected to an underwater seal and suction performed until pleural fusion occurs. After this time, the drain may be cut short and slowly removed in the manner of an empyema drain, even if the air leak continues.

The surgeon looking after the patient with a pneumothorax responding only slowly to drainage comes under a lot of pressure from the patient and from physicians. The patient is usually impatient to get the drain out and be mobile again, and needs much mental and physical support to accept a prolonged treatment. Physicians faced with a patient who is still losing air from a chest drain tend to be very gloomy and mention the words 'bronchopleural fistula', failing to recognize that all pneumothoraces occurring spontaneously are due to a bronchopleural fistula. The pressures for operative interference mount and the surgeon needs to retain patience and judgement. A sense of humour is essential when the drainage tube has been clamped in order to 'stop the bubbling', a treatment which is like plugging the rectum in order to stop diarrhoea.

Summary Chest drainage is needed after all thoracotomies in order to remove blood and secretions from the pleural cavity and to permit expansion of the lung. An underwater seal prevents air being introduced into the pleural cavity and all chest drains should be attached to suction.

Drains which are inserted to remove fluid should be left in place until the drainage is very low. The timing of removal of drains placed to remove air is more complex and is determined by the ability of the underlying lung to remain expanded. Frequent chest X-rays are essential in the management of chest drains.

Persisting controversies

- The desirability and amount of suction which should be applied to chest drains.
- The timing of removal of chest drains inserted to remove air.

Complications of the Chest Wall Incision

Nearly all lung operations are performed through a lateral thoracotomy. This incision is made with the patient lying on his opposite side, although some surgeons still prefer their patients in the face-down position. This prone position was used in the early days of pulmonary surgery when most operations were performed on patients with pulmonary tuberculosis who had excessive bronchial secretions. Nowadays, even in the minority of patients who have pulmonary tuberculosis, the prone position has been largely abandoned because secretions are less of a problem, mainly because of cuffed endobronchial or endotracheal tubes, earlier disease diagnosis and better physiotherapy.

The lateral incision may be extended anteriorly or posteriorly to afford better access (Fig. 2.10). The incision through the skin is placed so that it lies below the angle of the scapula and below the tissues of the breast. It is deepened through the bulky mass of the latissimus dorsi and the serratus anterior muscles. The rib cage is opened through the sixth intercostal space since good access is given to the hilum of the lung. Some surgeons remove a rib to improve the access even further.

Infection

Prevention. Obviously careful preparation of the skin before

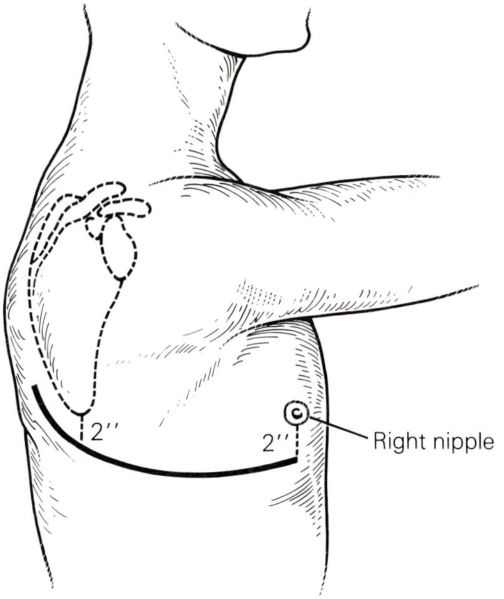

Figure 2.10
Skin incision for a lateral thoracotomy. This incision may be extended anteriorly or posteriorly if necessary.

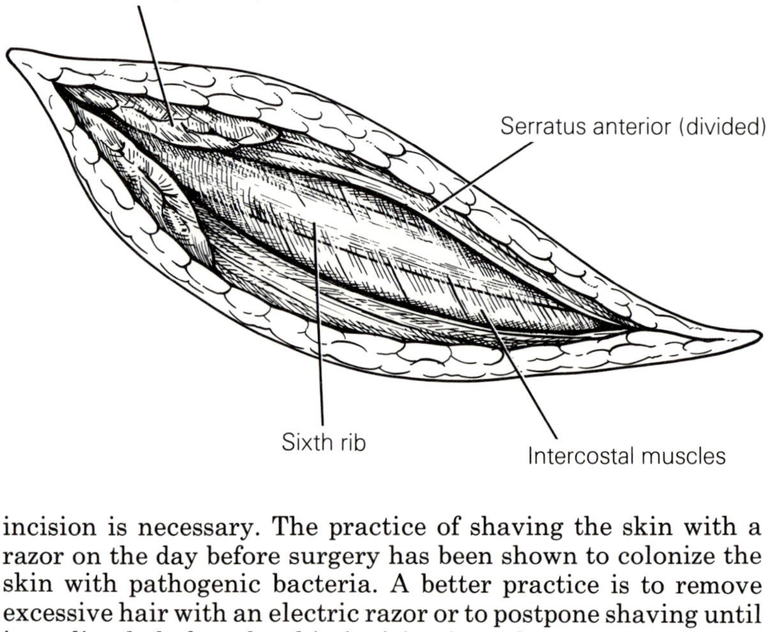

incision is necessary. The practice of shaving the skin with a razor on the day before surgery has been shown to colonize the skin with pathogenic bacteria. A better practice is to remove excessive hair with an electric razor or to postpone shaving until immediately before the skin incision is made.

The skin and subcutaneous tissue of the chest wall posteriorly is relatively avascular, tending to heal poorly and becoming easily infected. Infection may be reduced in this area by careful precise haemostasis and precise suturing, avoiding strangulation of the tissue afterwards.

Infection occurs in any wound where conditions allow the inevitable bacterial contamination to become established. In performing the chest incision, therefore, the surgeon should avoid damaging the tissue unduly by over-use of diathermy cautery by excessive traction and by a suturing technique which causes impairment of the blood supply.

Diagnosis. After operation, daily inspection of the wound usually reveals some inflammation, especially posteriorly. Undue swelling or cellulitis should lead to the sutures in the area being removed as underlying pus is probably present. Obviously any pus found should be examined in the bacteriology laboratory.

Treatment. The best treatment is to avoid the problem and careful surgical technique will go a long way towards this goal. Infection when diagnosed should be treated by drainage given by removal of sutures in both the skin and muscle layers as appropriate. Antibiotics are given as indicated by the sensitivity of the organisms found in the wound, but only when signs of a cellulitis are present or the patient is showing signs of a systemic reaction to the infection, such as a pyrexia or an elevated white cell count. To treat a well-contained pocket of pus which has subsequently been drained with a course of antibiotics is useless at best.

Once an infected wound has been opened and drained, it may be allowed to heal by secondary intention or occasionally it may be resutured when clean. Resuturing is rarely necessary, however, since the open thoracotomy wound tends to fall together very quickly. Occasionally, the entire thoracotomy wound may fall apart because of infection, exposing the underlying lung. The lung always remains fully expanded because of pleural fusion and no particular action is necessary. However, if the pleural cavity is empty, the situation is much more serious since the cavity will inevitably lead to persistence of the infection. Under these circumstances, the problem should be treated as a post-pneumonectomy empyema.

Haematoma of the chest incision

Prevention. The muscles of the chest wall are quite vascular and careful haemostasis is necessary when opening and closing the chest wall. Most thoracic surgeons use diathermy cautery when dividing the muscles, but larger vessels should be individually ligated.

Diagnosis. A haematoma of the chest wall may mimic and indeed may progress to an abscess. Tenderness and swelling should arouse suspicion. Fluctuation may be difficult to detect if the collection is deeply situated.

Treatment. Again, careful operative techniques will help to avoid this problem. Once established, however, a haematoma needs drainage. Simple needle aspiration is rarely effective and effective drainage is achieved by opening the affected part of the wound.

Pain in the chest incision

Some discomfort is inevitable after performing a thoracotomy and that occurring early should be treated as already described in this chapter. However, late discomfort is fairly common, particularly with the thoracotomy made lower than usual.

Prevention. Severe pain and discomfort late after thoracotomy is usually due to nerve damage. The neurovascular intercostal bundle runs immediately under the rib and the intercostal opening should be made by approaching the pleural cavity above a rib. When closing the chest wall, the rib cage should be sewn up in such a way as to avoid the intercostal bundles.

Diagnosis. Undue discomfort long after a thoracotomy may be due to the original disease involving the chest wall. The diagnosis of postoperative pain is made by exclusion of other causes.

Treatment. The pain occurring late after a thoracotomy is one of the most difficult problems to treat effectively. Many months may pass before it resolves spontaneously and during that time analgesics are required. Severe pain may be treated by specialized techniques of pain control now available in pain clinics, but frequent regular oral analgesic therapy remains the best treatment.

Summary

Most lung surgery is performed through a posterolateral thoracotomy which enters the chest through the fifth intercostal space. Infection and haematoma formation may be very difficult to detect in the deeply situated tissues with this incision. Pain in the incision may persist for a long time. Careful techniques will help to avoid most of these complications. Prolonged incisional pain may be very difficult to treat.

Complications of Pneumonectomy

Operative complications

Haemorrhage Intraoperative haemorrhage while performing a pneumonectomy remains the major technical hazard. Bleeding occurs from the major pulmonary artery and veins at the hilum of the lung or from other smaller vessels in the hilum, pulmonary ligament or chest wall.

Major vessel haemorrhage. The pulmonary artery and veins are thin and contain blood at low pressures, yet are, by reason of their flow, very large. Control, ligation and division of these vessels presents technical problems if a life-threatening haemorrhage is to be avoided.

1 *Control* of the vessels is achieved by extensive dissection in the plane *immediately* adjacent to the vessel wall. The length of vessel dissected is important and should include the main vessel and its first main branches. The beginner in lung surgery invariably dissects out too short a length of vessel to allow adequate control.
2 *Ligation* of the vessels may be performed without prior clamping because of their low pressure (Fig. 2.11). Thick non-absorbable ligatures are used and the aim is to place two proximal ligatures on the main vessel, one of which may transfix the vessel wall. Distal to these ligatures, there must be an adequate (1.5 times the diameter of the vessel) length of tissue, preferably of greater bulk than the proximal ligated vessel. Figure 2.11 shows the way of achieving this state. Distal ligatures are placed on the vessel to stop troublesome leakage of blood from the lung which is to be removed.
   The ligatures should be tied under a tension which will stop bleeding but yet not damage the vessel wall. While being tied, the vessel should not be under traction.
3 *Division* of the vessel is then performed leaving a stump of about 1.5 times the original diameter of the vessel distal to the proximal two ligatures.

Careful technique will avoid haemorrhage. If bleeding does occur, it will do so for the following avoidable reasons:

1 The vessel has been inadequately dissected and insufficient length obtained peripherally to allow adequate control. Such dissection is usually possible but central extension of a lung neoplasm may prevent it. In these circumstances, an adequate length of vessel may be obtained by opening the pericardium and dissecting centrally.
2 The ligatures cut the vessel wall by being tied too tightly.
3 The vessel is ligated under traction resulting in a ligature which loosens when the tension is decreased.
4 During division of the vessel, an inadequate proximal stump of insufficient bulk is left and the ligatures slip off.

If a major vessel haemorrhage does occur, finger pressure is usually enough to obtain temporary control. If the vessel has been adequately dissected, a controlling clamp may then be applied. If dissection has not been performed, an atraumatic vascular clamp may be placed aross the entire pulmonary hilum.

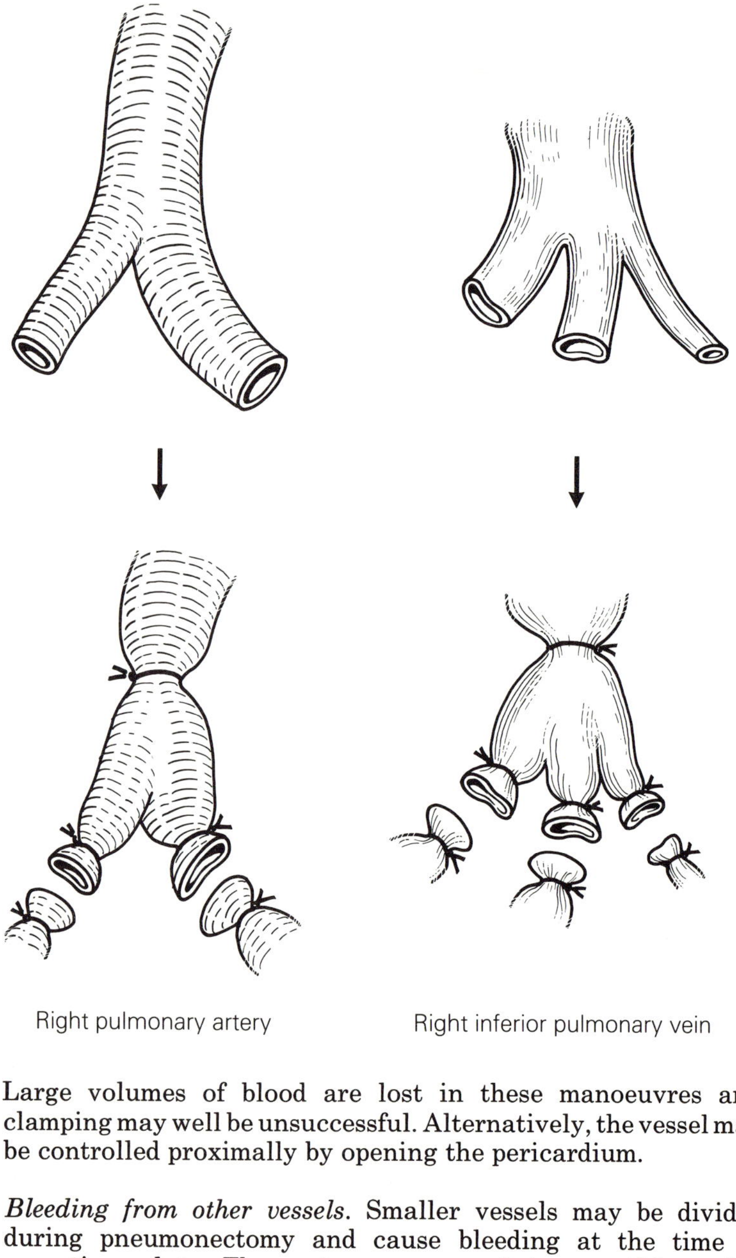

Figure 2.11
One method of safely ligating and dividing the pulmonary vessels.

Large volumes of blood are lost in these manoeuvres and clamping may well be unsuccessful. Alternatively, the vessel may be controlled proximally by opening the pericardium.

Bleeding from other vessels. Smaller vessels may be divided during pneumonectomy and cause bleeding at the time of operation or later. The most common vessels to cause this trouble are bronchial arteries in the peribronchial tissues or pulmonary ligament, or the intercostal arteries of the chest wall. Rarely, the lower lobe may be 'sequestrated' in that its blood supply arises not from the pulmonary circulation but by a large artery from the systemic circulation, usually the descending aorta. That vessel may be divided during pneumonectomy.

The bleeding from these vessels is usually visible at the time and easily stopped. If diathermy coagulation rather than ligation is used, however, bleeding will probably recur later. Therefore all vessels such as bronchial and intercostal arteries should be ligated individually rather than diathermied.

Damage to other structures

Damage to non-pulmonary structures during pneumonectomy usually occurs as a result of attempting to remove a lung lesion, such as bronchial carcinoma, which invades these structures. The experienced operating surgeon will often abandon pneumonectomy when faced with a problem which the less experienced will attempt to remove. No structure in the chest is immune from such damage. The heart and oesophagus may be damaged and the recurrent laryngeal nerve and thoracic duct divided. Growth may invade the superior vena cava and damage to this structure usually leads to fatal haemorrhage. Strangely, growth very rarely penetrates the aorta and may usually be cleanly removed from this structure without fear of haemorrhage.

Damage to the oesophagus may occur as a result of diathermy to the mediastinum.

Postoperative complications of pneumonectomy

In addition to respiratory failure and bronchopleural fistula (both discussed above) the empty hemithorax remaining after removal of the lung may cause complications in two ways. First, as in any other pathological cavity within the body, bacterial contamination is encouraged to cause active infection and a postoperative empyema may be caused. Second, the accumulation of air and blood in the hemithorax may disturb the position of the mediastinum and cause disturbance to the remaining lung.

Post-pneumonectomy empyema

Bacterial contamination is possible during the surgical operation or it may arise as an extension of infection in the chest wall. Commonly, the source of infection is a very small bronchopleural fistula.

Diagnosis. Symptoms of malaise occur usually within two weeks of pneumonectomy, but some patients may only become ill when convalescing at home. Examination usually shows a pyrexia and investigations show a polymorphonuclear leucocytosis. The chest X-ray is rarely very helpful. Confirmation of the diagnosis is made by needle aspiration and culture of fluid from the empty hemithorax.

Treatment. Drainage is essential. In patients who are very ill, insertion of an intercostal drainage tube under local anaesthesia will produce considerable improvement. Usually, it is not possible to get adequate dependent drainage through an intercostal tube no matter what its calibre is. Therefore, as soon as the condition of the patient permits, a *fenestration operation* must be performed.

The purpose of a fenestration is to form a large communication between the empyema space and the exterior so that free dependent drainage may occur. The body has remarkable powers of closing such holes spontaneously and the operation must take this into account. A lateral thoracotomy is made and at least 10 cm portions of the four ribs at the lowest part of the cavity are removed together with the intercostal muscles and overlying muscles of the trunk. The skin edges are then loosely sutured to the thickened parietal pleura. The result is a large hole in the chest wall through which it is possible to view most of the empyema cavity.

After the operation, the patient is encouraged to mobilize as soon as possible to allow drainage into a thick dressing. Many units irrigate the cavity with a variety of solutions, ranging from normal saline to antiseptic solutions, but it must be recognized that these are less important than adequate drainage.

Over the weeks that follow, the fenestration usually reduces in size by about two-thirds and the amount of drainage slowly reduces. Frequent bacteriological examination of the discharge will show that the original pathogens are replaced with a variety of 'non-pathogenic' organisms during this time. This period of treatment may be carried out either in hospital or at home if an adequate home nursing service is available.

Eventually, the interior of the chest will show granulation tissue only and no slough. This point may be reached quickly (in say six weeks) or slowly (perhaps six months). At this time, the cavity may be so small that spontaneous healing will follow. Usually, however, further surgery is needed. This consists of filling the chest with a weak solution of neomycin in saline (0.25%) and then closing the fenestration by forming a flap of skin and trunk muscle. By this stage, any bronchopleural fistula which may have been present originally has usually healed but occasionally a separate trimming of the bronchus and resuturing may be needed.

Postpneumonectomy empyema is a serious complication. Prevention by a careful surgical technique will reduce its incidence. Once established, however, successful treatment will often take months and the patient will need maximal physical and mental support.

Disturbances to the remaining lung after pneumonectomy

When the hemithorax becomes obliterated by fibrous tissue, and no cavity remains on the operated side, no further problems will arise. By this stage there is contraction of the chest wall, elevation of the diaphragm and some deviation of the mediastinum towards the operated side.

Until this stage is arrived at, however, complications may occur because of variations in the amount of blood and air in the empty hemithorax. If there is too much or too little air or fluid in the hemithorax, the mediastinum will shift either away from or towards the operated side. This, in itself, is not very important but the degree of compression or distension of the remaining lung is the reason why its function may become seriously diminished. The X-rays (Figs 2.12, 2.13) show the ideal position of the mediastinum after pneumonectomy. Using comparable films, the distance of the outer edge of the mediastinum from the chest wall on the side opposite to that of the operation is the same as, or slightly greater than, the distance before operation. This measurement is repeatedly made, using a ruler, on the films that are taken after surgery, always using the preoperative film as a comparison.

Many surgeons who have performed a pneumonectomy prefer to drain the chest for 24 hours. Others do not. Provided the mediastinum is maintained in a proper position, the means by which this is accomplished are unimportant.

If the chest is drained for 24 hours, the drain is clamped most of the time and unclamped for two minutes every hour. This allows any increased pressure within the empty hemithorax to be released and thus allows the mediastinum to remain central. After the drain is removed, however, the mediastinum does not become immobile and the pressure within the empty hemithorax

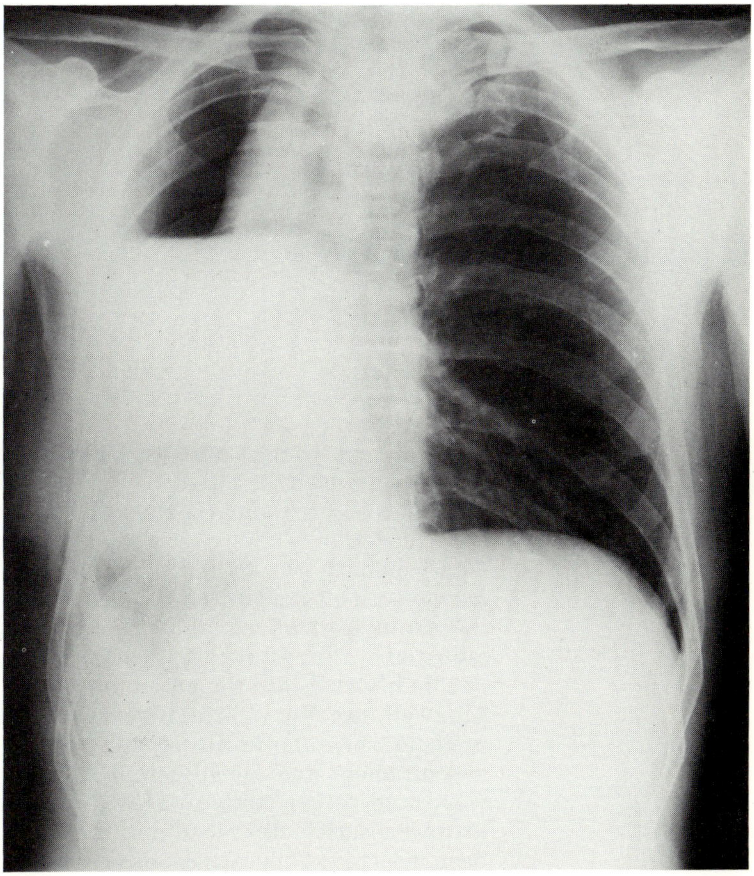

Figure 2.12 Chest X-ray of a normal right pneumonectomy. Note wedge shape of negative pressure air space and ipsilateral movement of mediastinum.

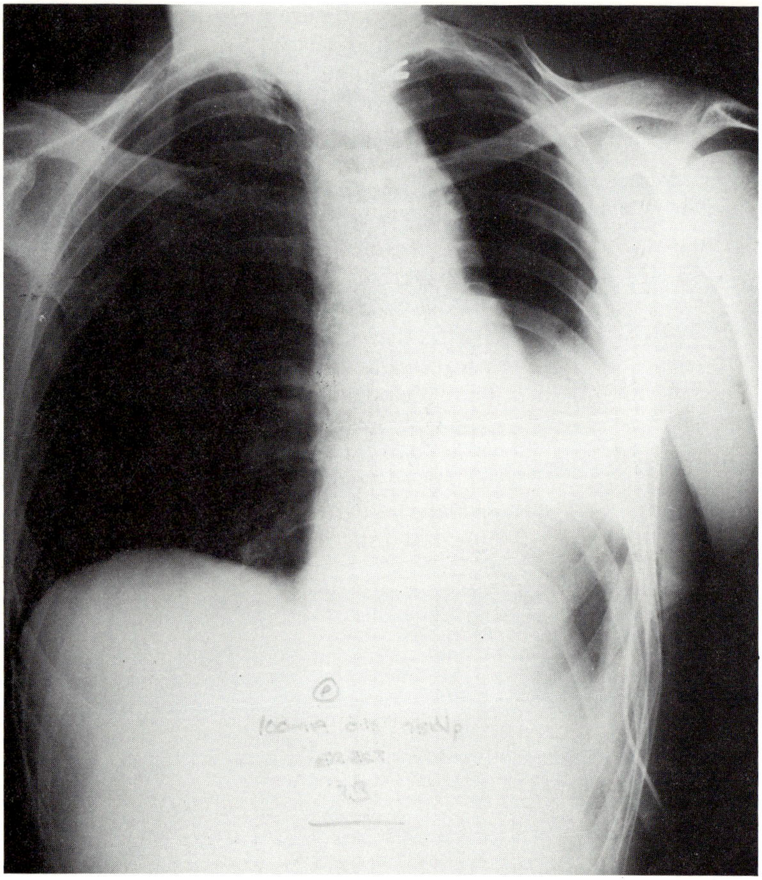

Figure 2.13
Chest X-ray of normal left pneumonectomy. Note the shift of the mediastinum to the operated side and triangular shape of the air space.

may vary, pushing it one way or another. Provided the mediastinum remains in the ideal position – detected clinically by slight deviation of the trachea to the operated side and radiologically as described above – there is no need to check the pressure in the empty hemithorax (which should be about −5 to −15 mHg). However, if clinical or radiological mediastinal shift occurs after the drain is removed, the pressures should be measured and adjusted by the removal or insertion of air. This is done by using a needle inserted into the pneumonectomy space connected to the Maxwell box (Fig. 2.14). This was originally designed to induce artificial pneumothoraces, and allows intrapleural pressure measurement and air adjustment to be performed. In a similar way, fluid rather than air may have to be removed in order to achieve a satisfactory mediastinal position. If no chest drain has been inserted at operation, the pressures must be checked at least

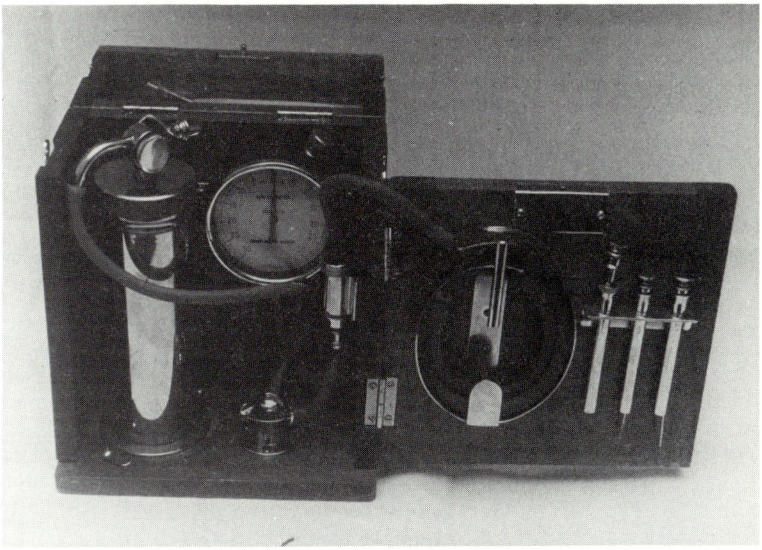

Figure 2.14
The Maxwell box. The graduated cylinder on the left allows removal or introduction of precise volumes of air.

three times in the first 24 hours and adjustments made by removal of air and/or fluid.

Usually, the mediastinum becomes deviated away from the operated side by an increased pressure caused by the accumulation of blood. This results in compression of the remaining lung (see Fig. 2.7). The resulting impaired function shows itself in various ways. The commonest is for the patient to be unduly short of breath and for the chest X-ray to show changes compatible with 'bronchopneumonia'. The sudden onset of atrial fibrillation or confusion may indicate arterial hypoxia. Frank respiratory failure with tachypnoea, drowsiness and sweating may follow. The diagnosis is made on the clinical and radiological criteria already described and the treatment is to reduce the elevated pressure on the operated side by removal of blood or fluid from the operated side. Supportive treatment, such as oxygen, digoxin therapy and ventilation, is important but secondary to correction of the underlying problem.

Much less commonly, the pressure on the operated side may be below 'normal' and this is usually due to a failure of fluid to accumulate in the empty space. The mediastinum is deviated towards the operated side and over-distension of the remaining lung occurs. The patient becomes uncomfortable rather than distressed and is relieved by air being introduced into the empty cavity by the Maxwell box. This situation usually resolves itself over a period of weeks, but every surgeon has one or two patients who have a 'dry' pneumonectomy space for years and who need to attend the hospital frequently so that air may be introduced into the chest.

Summary
The performance of pneumonectomy is attended by the problems of control of large, low-pressure thin-walled vessels. Haemorrhage may occur from bronchial or intercostal arteries. After operation, complications may arise from respiratory failure, bronchopleural fistula, postpneumonectomy empyema or from inadequate care of the pneumonectomy space.

Persisting controversy
- The necessity for chest drainage after pneumonectomy.

Postoperative complications after lobectomy

After lobectomy, the remaining lobes of the lung expand and this expansion, coupled with some mediastinal and diaphragmatic shift, leads to obliteration of any space on the operated side. Thus certain problems found after pneumonectomy become less important after lobectomy (Table 2.1).

Respiratory failure. This may occur after lobectomy and is detected and treated as described previously. Most patients after lobectomy show very little disturbance of respiratory function clinically because the lobectomy has been performed on anatomical criteria in that lobectomy was sufficient to adequately remove the disease.

Respiratory failure may occur, however, if the lobectomy has been performed on the physiological ground of preserving as much poorly functioning lung as possible. 'This patient will tolerate a lobectomy, but not a pneumonectomy' is a phrase which should arouse suspicion in any surgeon about to perform lung resection. One major reason is that respiratory function will show a temporary reduction much more than that which is to be expected from the removal of one lobe. Handling, surgical trauma and chest-wall pain all lead to diminished function in the remaining lobes and this, although temporary, may be enough to cause serious problems while it exists.

Bronchopleural fistula. This complication occurs infrequently after lobectomy because the peripheral bronchi tend to heal securely after division and suture. When a bronchopleural fistula does occur, however, it poses much less of a problem than after pneumonectomy, *provided the remaining lung remains fully*

Table 2.1
Postoperative complications after lobectomy.

1	Respiratory failure
2	Bronchopleural fistula
3	Persisting air leak
4	Failure of remaining lobes to expand

expanded and no empty space occurs in the hemithorax of the operated side. This will occur if the air entering the pleural space is removed at a faster rate than the rate at which it enters. After a week or two, the pleural cavity will become obliterated by fibrous fusion of the pleural layers. When this has occurred, the drainage tube may be removed from suction. If the remaining lung remains fully expanded on check X-rays, the tube may be removed slowly as in the manner of an empyema. However, if the air leak through the fistula is so great that the remaining lung collapses (and bronchial obstruction is ruled out by bronchoscopy), early surgical closure of the open fistula should be performed.

Persisting air leak. As stated previously, this is only rarely due to a bronchopleural fistula through the broken down lobar bronchus, and most commonly from the parenchyma of the remaining lobe. The distinction between the two is very difficult and of no practical significance, provided the remaining lung remains fully expanded. Treatment is exactly on the same grounds as outlined for bronchopleural fistula after lobectomy.

However, appropriate surgical techniques will reduce the amount of parenchymal leak occurring after lobectomy. The leaks usually come from damage inflicted in removing a lobe which has a poorly developed fissure separating it from its neighbour. Just as a meticulous careful dissection of the main bronchus will encourage poor healing, the meticulous dissection of a poorly developed fissure will cause undue laceration of the remaining lung in lobectomy.

When all the vessels and bronchus supplying the lobe to be removed are divided, and the remaining lung inflated by the anaesthetist, firm traction on the distal bronchus and counter-traction with a swab on the remaining lung will result in the lobe being removed along the true fissure. This technique looks and is crude. Nevertheless, it is effective and reduces air leakage from the remaining lung.

Two drainage tubes, one apical and one basal, should always be used after lobectomy. The basal tube is usually quickly removed when fluid stops draining. The apical tube is left in for 24 hours after the last air bubble has been seen. If the lung remains fully expanded, the drain is then clamped overnight. If the lung is seen to be fully expanded on an X-ray the next morning, the apical tube may then be safely removed.

Failure of the remaining lobes to expand

1 *Operative causes.* Failure to mobilize the lung properly, and in particular to divide the pulmonary ligament fully, will lead to a tendency of the remaining lobes to expand poorly. The remedy is clear. Undue mobility of a segment of lung adjacent to a larger lobe (e.g. the lingula) may lead to its twisting and strangulation. Such a situation may be avoided by tacking the

smaller mobile lobe to the larger with a few interrupted sutures.

2 *Postoperative causes.* Extensive contusion of a remaining lobe will make it stiff and less likely to expand fully but most cases of failure of a lobe to expand are due to bronchial obstruction. Only rarely, as in the case of a surgical bronchopleural fistula, are the drainage tubes inadequate. Bronchoscopy and removal of the secretions in the bronchial tree will permit aeration and expansion. This bronchoscopy should be performed on the ward under local and topical anaesthesia since the patient's co-operation in deep breathing will improve the result. Similarly, a physiotherapist may mobilize secretions from the peripheral bronchi which would otherwise be inaccessible to bronchoscopic suction.

Summary. The complications of lobectomy are much less serious than those occurring after pneumonectomy. Provided adequate drainage allows full expansion of the remaining lung, infection and bronchopleural fistula are easily treated.

Complications of Other Lung Operations

Segmentectomy

Removal of a bronchopulmonary segment of a lobe is occasionally practised for excision of a very localized disease. The complications are in all ways similar to those following lobectomy and the same principles of treatment apply. Surgical technique is very important in segmentectomy so that the pulmonary vessels and bronchus specific to that segment are identified precisely before any structure is divided. This means in practice that all the vessels and bronchi of a particular lobe have to be dissected meticulously before accurate identification is possible. The vascular anatomy may vary and no assumptions should be made without all the structures being visible. Removal of a segment from the surrounding lung parenchyma is difficult unless the procedure described for lobectomy with a poorly developed fissure is followed. Contusion of the remaining lung is usually quite severe, causing an impressive shadowing on the chest X-ray which may last for some months. Provided this is not infected, and the lung fully fits the hemithorax, no action is needed.

Removal of lung 'cysts'

Lung cysts occur in infancy and later in life. Because of their size and tension, they may cause compression of the remaining lung on the same side, deviation of the mediastinum and compression of the opposite lung. Thus surgery is performed in order to remove the cyst or to reduce its size and tension to a level which allows the remaining lung tissue to work properly.

Lung cysts in children

Large spaces under tension may result from accessory lung tissue, accessory bronchial tissue, staphylococcal infection and congenital lobar emphysema. Although each has a different cause, their effects are the same and removal of the cyst is usually accomplished by lobectomy. This leaves behind healthy lung which expands and functions normally. No specific complications arise.

Lung cysts in adults

These cysts are usually emphysematous in origin and represent the coalescence of several smaller areas of emphysema. Clearly, the rest of the lungs will be damaged to a lesser degree and this makes the decision to operate much less clear cut than in children, because it may not be clear which lesion is imposing the greater disability. In general terms, most surgeons will only operate on degenerative lung cysts if the cysts are bigger than one-third of the volume of the hemithorax and if there is clear clinical, radiographic and spirometric evidence that the patient's disability is caused by the cyst.

The surgical operation takes into account the background of chronic lung disease and is as limited as possible. A simple deroofing of the largest cyst is performed and the walls of the cyst approximated by interrupted or continuous catgut sutures. Remaining disease in the lung or lobe is ignored.

After the operation, there may be a prolonged air leak for some weeks which should be managed as already described. During this time, those attending the patient should be aware of the possibility of a pneumothorax developing on the opposite side and equipment should be available to allow insertion of a chest drain at short notice.

Further reading

(for Complications of Pulmonary Surgical Investigations)

Block, A.J. & Olson, G.N. (1976) Preoperative pulmonary function testing. *JAMA, 235*, 257.

Boyd, A.D. & Spencer, F.C. (1983) Endoscopy: bronchoscopy and esophagoscopy. In: *Gibbons Surgery of the Chest*, ed. D.C. Sabiston Jr & F.C. Spencer, 4th edn, vol. 1. Philadelphia: W.B. Saunders.

Brock, R.C. (1954) *The Anatomy of the Bronchial Tree*. London: Oxford University Press.

Fraser, R. & Paré, J.A.P. (1977–1979) *Diagnosis of Diseases of the Chest*, vols 1–4. Philadelphia: W.B. Saunders.

Heaston, D.K., Mills, S.R., Moore, A.V. & Johnston, W.W. (1981) Percutaneous thoracic needle biopsy. In: *Pulmonary Diagnosis*, ed. E.C. Putnam. New York: Appleton-Century-Crofts.

Pearson, F.G. (1968) An evaluation of mediastinoscopy in the management of presumably operable bronchial carcinoma. *J. Thorac. Cardiovasc. Surg., 55*, 617.

Sarin, C.L. & Nohl Osler, H.C. (1969) Mediastinoscopy. *Thorax, 24*, 585.

Saunders, R.D. (1967) The ventilating attachments for bronchoscopy. *Del. Med. J.*, *39*, 170.

(for Complications of Pulmonary Operations and Chest Wall Incision)

Barker, W.L., Faber, L.P., Ostermuller, W.E. & Langstone, H.T. (1971) Management of persistent bronchopleural fistulas. *J. Thorac. Cardiovasc. Surg.*, *62*, 393.

Belcher, J.R. & Sturridge, M.F. (1972) *Thoracic Surgical Management*, 4th edn. London: Baillière Tindall.

Forrester-Wood, C.P. (1980) Bronchopleural fistula following pneumonectomy for carcinoma of the bronchus. *J. Thorac. Cardiovasc. Surg.*, *80*, 400.

Goldstraw, P. (1970) Treatment of post pneumonectomy empyema: the case for fenestration. *Thorax*, *34*, 740.

Johnson, J., MacVaugh, H. & Waldhansen, J.A. (1973) *Surgery of the Chest*, 4th edn. Chicago: Year Book Medical Publishers.

3 Complications of Surgery to the Chest Wall and Diaphragm

All intrathoracic operations require the chest to be opened by one means or another, but there is also a group of conditions of the chest wall and diaphragm which require surgical solutions and therefore carry the risk of complications. It is these which will be considered in this chapter.

Regardless of the nature of the operation, chest wall and diaphragmatic operations heal well and no special precautions have to be observed from this aspect.

Haematoma of the chest wall operation is common because of the bulk and vascular nature of the trunk muscles. Often the haematoma lies very deep between the bony rib cage and the overlying muscles, and may be difficult to detect unless there is an awareness of its possible presence. Persisting discomfort and tenderness in the operative site should suggest a haematoma, but fluctuation is a late and unreliable sign. The complication can be largely prevented by careful haemostasis at the time of the original operation and most surgeons use diathermy cautery freely at this time.

Small tube suction drainage (e.g. 'Redivac') will prevent haematoma in susceptible wounds and thus reduce the possibility of infection. Once a haematoma is suspected, it should be aspirated via a wide bore needle or removed at a separate second operation.

Diaphragmatic incisions may damage the nerve supply to the diaphragm and result in partial or complete paralysis (Fig. 3.1). Analysis of the pattern of nerve supply to the diaphragm has yielded consistent results. As Fig. 3.1. shows, most of the nerve supply emanates from the phrenic nerve which passes down the mediastinum and pericardium to reach the diaphragm just medial to the dome of the diaphragm. The branches then pass in a series of loops to all but the most peripheral 5 cm of the diaphragm. This area is supplied by the nerves of the adjacent chest wall (intercostal nerves). Incisions in the diaphragm should therefore be placed circumferentially about 5 cm away from the

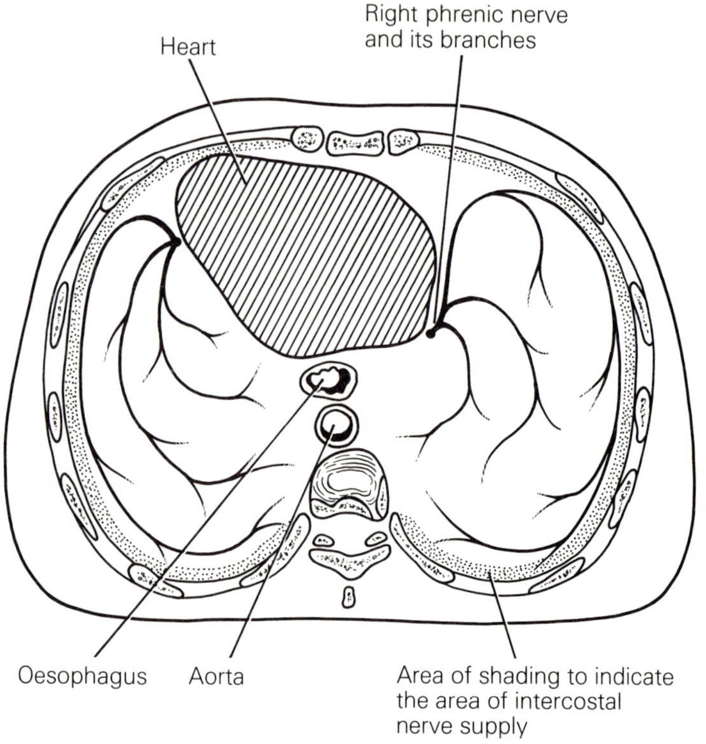

Figure 3.1 Pattern of innervation of the diaphragm.

chest wall. The traditional radial incision in the diaphragm will inevitably cause some nervous damage and subsequent paralysis.

There are four major types of chest wall operation: (a) operations for correction of deformity; (b) operations for removal of chest wall tumours; (c) thoracoplasty operations; and (d) the median sternotomy.

Operations for Correction of Deformity

Deformity of the pattern of sternal and adjacent costal cartilage growth results in either undue bowing anteriorly of the sternum (pectus carinatum) or undue depression of the sternum (pectus excavatum). Neither type of deformity causes derangement of intrathoracic physiology but the cosmetic effects of the abnormality may be quite striking. The surgeon is requested to correct the deformity in more severe cases.

The principle of the operation is common to both types of lesion. The sternum is mobilized by division or excision of the costal cartilages and by transverse fracture of the sternomanubrial junction. Using a variety of techniques, the sternum is then rigidly held in its correct position. Possibly the most preferred technique at the present time is to rest the sternum on Steinmann pins passed from the ribs on either side through the medulla of the sternum. When sound healing has occurred, the pins are removed at a second operation.

Complications
The major complication is that the operation may fail to correct the deformity which recurs in the months or years following the operation. Only wide excision of the deformed costal cartilages will help to prevent this. Nevertheless, there is always the possibility of this complication, and it is prudent to forewarn patients before surgery is performed.

Infection is the other major complication and is dealt with on page 31. The situation is, of course, complicated by the presence of the foreign bodies on the Steinmann pins and is unlikely to respond to conventional treatment until the pins are removed.

Respiratory failure may occur as a result of the 'flail segment' of the sternum. In some patients, some form of chest wall splinting may be omitted during the operation because the surgeon judged that the 'flail sternum' will not compromise the mechanical efficiency of the chest wall. In children, this judgement is very often correct, but becomes more difficult as the patients approach adult life. Respiratory failure often occurs on the third or fourth postoperative day and is diagnosed on clinical and laboratory grounds. When present, respiratory failure is treated by prolonged mechanical ventilation until sound healing of the bony chest wall occurs. This may take three to four weeks and the patient may be made more comfortable if a tracheostomy is performed. The ventilation provides internal splinting of the flail segment. Direct splinting of the sternum at this stage is usually ineffective and often leads to infection.

Operations for Removal of Chest Wall Tumours

Most tumours of the chest wall are either metastatic or occur as a result of direct extension from other organs such as the lung.

Removal of chest wall tumours is performed when such tumours become painful or, rarely, when the tumour is a primary one. In either case, the tumour is removed along with adjacent ribs, neurovascular bundles and associated muscles. A defect in the chest wall is created and obviously this will be covered over by skin and subcutaneous tissue during closure of the operative wound. This repair will be 'flail' and depending on its size will cause inefficiency of ventilation, perhaps leading to respiratory failure. If the segment to be removed is larger than 10 cm in diameter, it is usually necessary to attempt the insertion of a rigid plate within the repair to prevent flail. These are all foreign bodies, however, and any bacterial contamination will inevitably progress to infection. The operation is therefore conducted with meticulous technique and, should infection occur, early removal of the splint should be performed. Afterwards, the patient will need to be ventilated until the healing of the chest wall is rigid enough to permit adequate spontaneous respiration.

Thoracoplasty Operations

Thoracoplasty is performed in order to obliterate cavities in the thorax within which chronic infection persists. The cavities are usually produced by tuberculosis and the very presence of a cavity makes tubercle bacilli persist in spite of what would normally be effective chemotherapy. Currently, in Europe at least, removal of the diseased lung is the commonest surgical solution and thoracoplasty is infrequently performed. However, some very ill patients may only be suitable for thoracoplasty or the facilities available may not permit thoracotomy and lung resection.

Thoracoplasty comprises removing the ribs of the chest wall and allowing it to fall inwards compressing and collapsing the diseased lung. If the cavity is very large, many ribs may have to be removed. A staged procedure is usually performed if more than four ribs have to be removed in order to prevent respiratory insufficiency. At the first operation the upper four ribs are removed, and the chest wall is then allowed to heal and fibrose for a period of weeks before any further ribs are removed.

The major complications are those of respiratory failure and wound infection, and these are dealt with as described above. The major *late* complication of thoracoplasty, however, is a progressive scoliotic deformity caused by the healing process in the collapsed chest. Attention to posture and physical exercise will prevent this but only if the treatment is started within a few days of the operation. Even with adequate physiotherapy, however, the loss of the convexity of the chest wall leads to unsightly deformity; this is one of the reasons why the operation is done much less frequently than in years past.

The Median Sternotomy

The median sternotomy incision defies all criteria but one of a good surgical incision. It is sited vertically on the midline anteriorly on the chest wall and passes through the chest by dividing the sternum longitudinally. It therefore has a tendency to heal poorly and to be unsightly. However, the major virtue of a median sternotomy is that it affords reasonable access to all parts of the heart and great vessels within the thorax and is therefore widely used in cardiac surgery. Many of the complications of the median sternotomy are avoidable by careful surgical technique. Complications of the incision are difficult to treat and cause prolonged morbidity and sometimes mortality.

Technique

The incision through the skin extends from the suprasternal notch to about 4 cm below the xiphisternum and is kept strictly to the midline. The incision is deepened down to the anterior periosteum of the sternum which is divided by diathermy. The sternum is then divided vertically by an electric saw, again keeping to the midline, and the two halves of the bone are retracted to allow diathermy of the bleeding points of the posterior periosteum.

Any deviation of the incision away from the midline will greatly increase bleeding since the pectoralis major muscle fibres will be divided. During the division of the bone, it is usual to deflate the lungs in order to prevent opening the right pleural cavity.

Diathermy should be used as sparingly as possible on specific bleeding points so as to reduce damage to the soft tissues and periosteum to a minimum. Bleeding from the medulla of the sternum is controlled by bone wax but again specific points of bleeding are treated individually rather than bone wax being generally used.

Closure of the median sternotomy is performed after a drain has been left in the anterior mediastinum. The bone is approximated by interrupted stainless steel wire sutures passed through rather than round the bone. At least five and preferably six sutures are needed to ensure a sound apposition of the bone in adults. The soft tissue layers are then closed separately (muscle, subcutaneous tissue and skin), using continuous suture of absorbable material such as catgut or Dexon. Particular attention is paid to the closure of the upper part of the rectus sheath and interrupted sutures may be used.

The above technique causes minimal tissue damage and prevents haematoma formation. Unabsorbable foreign bodies are reduced to a minimum by the sparing use of bone wax and absorbable sutures.

Early complications (Table 3.1)

Minor Many, if not most, median sternotomy wounds have a slight discharge about four to five days postoperatively. This discharge should be examined bacteriologically, but unless it is accom-

Table 3.1
Complications of median sternotomy.

Early	*Late*
Minor	*Minor*
Wound discharge	Painful incision
Wound inflammation	Persisting discharge
Major	*Major*
Sternal mobility	Failure of sternal union
Mediastinitis	

panied by cellulitis or a systemic reaction no antibiotic treatment is necessary.

Spreading wound inflammation superficial to the bone should be treated by antibiotics and superficial sutures removed to allow free drainage. As the opened wound improves, the temptation to perform secondary closure should be resisted.

Major Early sternal mobility may occur if the wires break or cut through the softened bones of the elderly or sick patient. The resulting mobility may be painful but not affect respiration, or it may be so great as to cause problems with coughing and breathing. Slight painful mobility may be expected to stabilize very rapidly over a few days and only analgesics are required.

Wide sternal disruption is usually associated with a discharge from the wound. The patient rapidly becomes ill from a combination of pulmonary and wound problems. When this happens, early reoperation is advised and effective apposition of the sternum is performed together with drainage of the anterior mediastinum.

If at operation the wires are broken, they are merely replaced, but if they have cut through the bone, a more complicated sternal closure must be performed (Fig. 3.2). Alternatively, the halves of the sternum may be approximated by the use of broad, flat, plastic bands placed around the bone.

The drain in the anterior mediastinum is left in place until the discharge ceases and is then slowly withdrawn, preferably with the aid of repeated sinograms.

In such a potentially infected wound, interrupted rather than running sutures should be used on the soft tissues and skin.

Mediastinitis. The distinction between a disrupted sternal wound and mediastinitis is not often very clear. Certainly, sternal mobility is usually present in mediastinitis and there is a profuse discharge from the wound. The patient becomes very toxic and systemically disturbed, with a high white cell count and pyrexia.

As with a disrupted sternum, early operation is performed. At that time, there will be signs of liquid pus and slough between the halves of the sternum and in the anterior mediastinum. Actual necrosis of the bony edges may have occurred.

A variety of treatments have been used for this condition. Many surgeons favour excision of all damaged and infected tissue, and closure of the chest wall over a drain. We, however, have taken a much more conservative approach. The wound is opened, either with or without an anaesthetic, and left open. The sternal halves are retracted laterally, exposing the anterior mediastinum which is allowed to drain freely. The subsequent healing by secondary intention may take weeks – not all in hospital. We have avoided the excision of tissue and anything other than the sparing use of antiseptic agents such as povidone-iodine. Mechanical ventilation may be required initially but the

Figure 3.2 One method of closing the sternum if simple closure is ineffective.

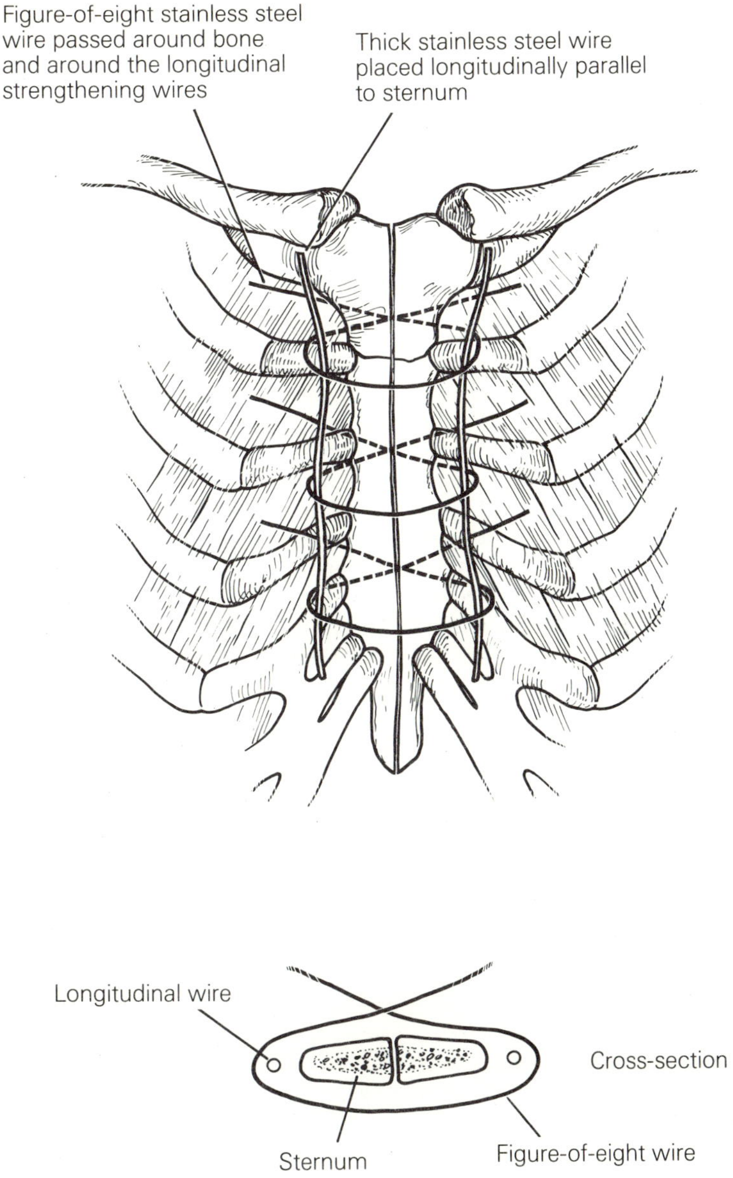

healing of the open wound is usually sufficiently rapid to allow spontaneous respiration fairly quickly. The open wound is surprisingly well tolerated by the patient and increasing activity should be permitted. When the wound needs dressing just once in the day, the patient is allowed home, provided that an adequate home nursing service is available. Once the solid slough in the wound separates, ultraviolet irradiation will encourage the rapid growth of granulation tissue. Such a wound will take from five to 12 weeks for full healing to occur.

Late complications (see Table 3.1)

Painful incision

Discomfort in a sternotomy wound is usually mild but some patients may have persisting discomfort for several weeks after their discharge from hospital. As long as there is no inflammation, undue mobility or systemic disturbance, reassurance and mild analgesics are effective. Examination of the wound may reveal areas of localized exquisite tenderness. These areas should be explored because there is usually a foreign body causing the discomfort. Sternal or pacemaker wires are the usual culprits. Frequently such wires are accompanied by a small discharging sinus. Again, the only effective treatment is to remove the wire. To culture the discharge and then treat with an appropriate antibiotic is rarely effective.

Painful wires can usually be removed under local anaesthetic. After a thorough infiltration of the local anaesthetic agent, a small transverse incision is made over the wire, cutting through the sinus if present. Granulation tissue is removed by curettage and the wire cut and removed. Gentle curettage of the underlying sternum helps to remove any small areas of dead bone and granulation tissue. The wound is loosely packed and allowed to heal by secondary intention. Antibiotics are not given routinely.

Failure of sternal union

Rarely, the sternotomy wound remains painful for some months or years after operation. Examination reveals slight sternal mobility which is painful. The sternal halves heal by a fibrous union under these circumstances. The treatment is operative and consists of reopening the wound and freshening the sternal edges. Tight and accurate apposition of the bone is then achieved by multiple interrupted stainless steel wire sutures.

Taking into consideration all the above, the vast majority of sternal wounds heal with great speed and with very little discomfort.

Summary

All thoracic operations involve operating on the chest wall. The incisions used in lung surgery carry the complications of any other wound. The median sternotomy is widely used in cardiac surgery and has a tendency to heal less well than lateral thoracotomy incisions. Operations on the chest wall itself usually involve removing a greater or lesser part of the rigid thoracic cage and may cause respiratory inefficiency. The amount of chest wall which can be removed without this complication varies, but is never more than about 10 cm in diameter. If more than this is removed, the chest wall defect must be made rigid by a prosthesis or the patient mechanically ventilated until the resulting scar is rigid enough to permit normal breathing.

Further reading

Alley, R.D. (1964) Thoracic surgical incisions and postoperative drainage. In: *The Craft of Surgery*, ed. P. Cooper, vol. 1. Boston: Little, Brown and Company.
Clagett, O.T. & Johnson, M.A., III (1949) Tumors of the diaphragm. *Am. J. Surg.*, *78,* 526.
Lees, W.M. (1983) Thoracic incisions. In: *General Thoracic Surgery*, ed. T.W. Shields. Philadelphia: Lea and Febiger.

4 Complications of Chest Injuries

The management of chest injuries is undertaken by many hospitals which do not have a specialized cardiothoracic surgical unit. Most of these injuries are treated very well, but in a number of cases complications arise and are referred on to a cardiothoracic unit for further treatment. There can be no doubt that some of these complications are avoidable if a specialized opinion is obtained initially, but equally many are unavoidable. The management of complications arising from chest injuries is demanding and usually involves close co-operation with other disciplines because most patients suffer multiple injuries. Since the ideal aim of management is to avoid complications, inevitably this chapter must be concerned with the initial handling of the injured patient because appropriate early treatment can in many cases avoid what may be a life-threatening series of complications.

Many patients with chest injuries also have other injuries to the trunk, head and limbs. Apart from severe bleeding occurring elsewhere, the management of the chest injury takes precedence over the management of other injuries because of the immediately life-threatening possibilities which arise. Deficiencies in the supply of oxygenated blood in the brain and myocardium are so rapidly fatal that other injuries must be ignored until the adequacy of cerebral and myocardial oxygenation is assured.

The nature of chest injuries. Chest injuries are either 'blunt' or 'penetrating'. In the United Kingdom, the majority of chest injuries arise from road accidents and are blunt. In other parts of the world, penetrating injuries arising from malice are more common but there is a trend in increasing numbers of penetrating injuries in the United Kingdom.

Death Without a Diagnosis

This is the major and most worrying complication of chest injury. Frequently, a multiple-injured patient arrives in the accident room in poor condition and dies within a few minutes while the attending surgeons are still trying to work out the nature of the injuries and what to do about them. The nature of hospital organization means that the most senior and experienced individuals are rarely available at these crucial moments and the heavy responsibilities fall on relatively inexperienced and unspecialized medical staff.

When a patient arrives in the hospital *in extremis* clinical history and examination are clearly inappropriate. A rapid, necessarily rather superficial, examination is needed. The chest should be uncovered and its movements observed. At the same time, the femoral or carotid pulse should be felt and the adequacy of ventilation assessed by listening to the passage of air in and out of the mouth.

If the sound of air passing into the patient appears adequate, it is likely that oxygenation and ventilation are, at least for the moment, satisfactory. If, on the other hand, the force or frequency of expired/inspired air is impaired, a significant ventilation problem exists.

Inspection of the chest wall will detect any differences in expansion and any 'flail' segment will be obvious. The rare event of an open pneumothorax will be obvious to inspection. Emergency intubation and positive-pressure ventilation should be started immediately. A poor quality femoral or carotid pulse almost certainly indicates a low cardiac output and probably oligaemia.

The next step is to palpate the neck, particularly noting the position of the trachea. Gross deviation of the trachea always indicates that there is a tension problem on the side of the chest from which the trachea is deviated. Whether the tension is due to blood or air is unimportant. What is important is the compression of the other lung caused by the mediastinal shift. In a patient who is dying from injuries, the presence of gross mediastinal shift should lead to the insertion of a chest drain *without X-ray control* into the hemithorax away from which the trachea has deviated.

If the trachea is not widely deviated and if the adequacy of ventilation and femoral pulses is satisfactory, the likelihood of the patient dying within a few minutes is remote. The attending surgeon may then proceed at a more leisurely pace to make a full clinical and radiological assessment and plan the treatment in an unhurried and rational manner.

Summary

A rapid screening examination is necessary when the patient with chest injuries arrives in the hospital in order to prevent death occurring shortly after arrival. The adequacy of ventilation and a major pulse should be assessed and the chest inspected. Gross tracheal deviation is an extreme emergency and should be treated by intercostal chest drainage, if necessary, without the benefit of a chest X-ray. If ventilation is inadequate, intubation and positive-pressure ventilation must be started. An inadequate major pulse indicates oligaemia and an infusion must be started.

Persisting controversies

- Insertion of chest drainage without the benefit of chest X-ray diagnosis.

- Emergency thoracotomy on patients who arrive clinically dead will result in some survivors.

Once the situation has been assessed and the probability of sudden death largely eliminated, a full examination is performed in the accident department. The colour of the patient is noted in a good light and the perfusion of the hands and feet noted. The neck is re-examined to detect any evidence of emphysema. Clinical examination of the chest will show any localized tenderness or flail segment, and auscultation will show any difference of breath sounds. Examination of the rest of the patient should follow, paying particular attention to the abdomen, limbs and cervical spine.

If the condition of the patient is stable, a chest X-ray should then be taken. Although the patient has injuries, every effort should be made to achieve a degree of head-up posture since haemothorax, in particular, may be missed on a film taken in the supine position.

If it is clear that the chest injury is anything other than minor, it is desirable at this stage to set up an intravenous infusion, to insert a urinary catheter and to insert a central venous line via the internal jugular vein. This latter cannulation allows measurement of the central venous pressure and, more importantly, access to the central circulation if needed. If the patient is breathing spontaneously, a face mask with added inspired oxygen will not do any harm and may be of benefit.

Complications of Blunt Chest Injuries

Fracture of the ribs

Any blunt injury to the chest may cause a fracture of one or more ribs. Multiple fractures of ribs do not necessarily produce an unstable chest wall or flail segment unless each rib is broken in two or more places.

Fractures of the ribs should always raise the suspicion of underlying visceral or arterial injury. Indeed, certain ribs – such as the first – are so protected that the degree of force necessary to fracture it is so great that intense suspicion should be aroused.

Rib fractures always heal and malunion is very rare. The major complication of a simple fracture is the intense pain which it causes. This pain restricts the depth of breathing and coughing and impairs the process of tracheobronchial toilet. As a consequence atelectasis and peneumonia may follow, and in older age groups this complication may prove fatal.

The traditional treatment of strapping the chest firmly in order to immobilize the fracture and thus lessen pain is now largely discredited. The degree of pain relief is inadequate and the immobilization of the chest wall often produces the complications which it is sought to avoid. Adequate pain relief can be obtained either by an intercostal block or by the direct injection of local anaesthetic into the fracture site. The relief from this latter procedure is surprisingly long in duration and usually only two or three injections are required. The complications of rib fracture, which will now be discussed, are listed in Table 4.1.

Pneumothorax

The sharp end of a fractured rib may penetrate the parietal and the visceral pleura and puncture the underlying lung. A pneumothorax will result and give rise to a typical X-ray picture. There is some residual controversy as to whether spontaneous pneumothoraces should be treated by drainage, but none at all concerning traumatic pneumothoraces because there can be no certainty that a simple traumatic pneumothorax will not progress rapidly to a tension pneumothorax. Therefore, any pneumothorax associated with an injury should be treated with an intercostal drain connected to an underwater seal and placed on suction (see Fig. 2.8). The ideal method of drain insertion has already been described (see pages 25–26).

Tension pneumothorax

When the pneumothorax develops a positive pressure and displaces the mediastinum to the opposite side, thus compressing the opposite lung, *tension* is said to exist and is a life-threatening condition. Urgent drainage is needed – preferably with X-ray control – but, as already described (see pages 24–25), under extreme circumstances the intercostal drain may have to be inserted on clinical grounds.

Haemothorax

In a similar manner, a haemothorax may arise as a consequence of a fractured rib and the condition may be simple or tension may be created (Fig. 4.1). In either case, intercostal drainage is indicated by the same criteria and by the same techniques as in pneumothorax.

There is usually a large loss of blood into the drainage bottle as the accumulated blood is drained. Thereafter, the drainage rapidly subsides as the underlying lung is expanded to the chest wall and lacerations compressed. However, sometimes bleeding will persist. If the amounts persistently stay above 500 ml/h for three or more consecutive hours, a thoracotomy is indicated. Thoracotomy may be necessary to remove clotted blood within the hemithorax since this will prevent full expansion of the underlying lung and will eventually organize and become a fibrothorax.

Table 4.1
Complications of rib fractures.

1 Pneumothorax
2 Tension pneumothorax
3 Haemothorax
4 Flail chest
5 Surgical emphysema

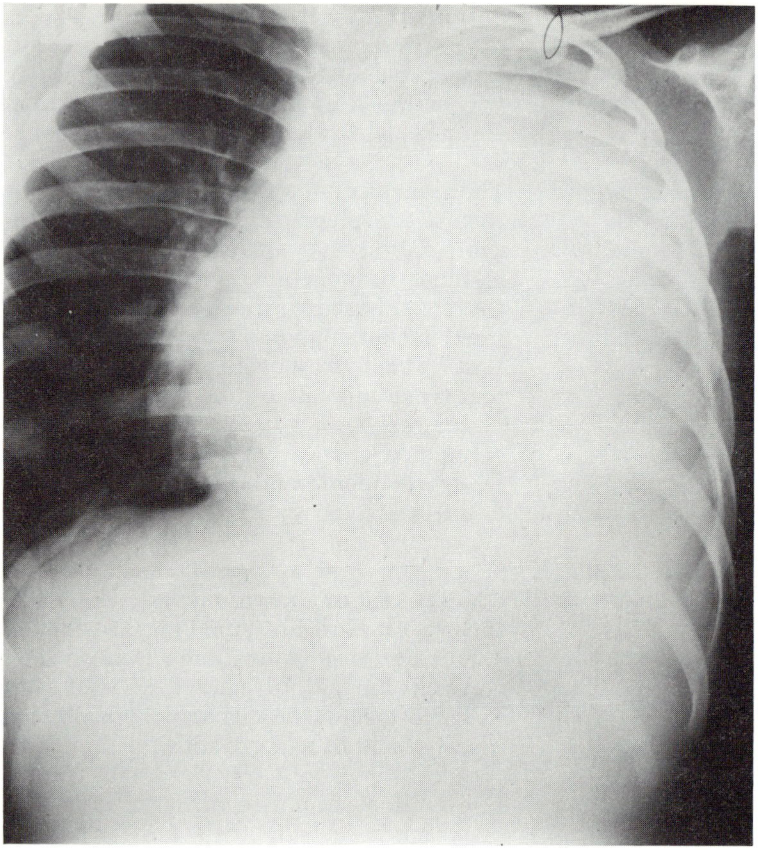

Figure 4.1
Chest X-ray of a large left haemothorax following a chest injury. Note shift to right of mediastinum causing compression of opposite lung (cf. Fig. 2.7).

As a general rule, the intercostal drain should be connected to suction. This may temporarily increase the bleeding, but as the lung tamponades against the chest wall bleeding will subside rapidly thereafter.

Flail chest If the rigidity of the chest wall is destroyed by fractures of the ribs or costal cartilages, a segment of the chest wall will move in on inspiration and out on expiration. This leads to considerable respiratory problems in ventilating the underlying lung. The size of the segment which will produce embarrassment depends on the fitness and age of the patient. A flail segment of 10–12 cm in diameter will cause problems in a fit adult, but in older patients or those with respiratory disease a much smaller segment may cause respiratory distress and, ultimately, failure.

Treatment. As a first-aid measure, the flail segment should be pushed into the chest and immobilized by a pressure pad. This will do the underlying lung no good whatsoever but will allow efficient ventilation of the opposite lung.

Later, the flail segment should be stabilized. Many attempts have been made to produce a reliable method of externally splinting the flail segment but a satisfactory solution has not been agreed upon. The most favoured way is to ensure stability and adequate ventilation by positive-pressure mechanical ventilation. This is achieved by an orotracheal tube or, later, a tracheostomy.

Small flail segments may become stable after a few days of ventilation. Larger segments usually require three weeks to allow the fractures sufficient healing time to restore the rigidity of the chest wall. Therefore, if a patient needs long-term ventilation, a tracheostomy should be performed at the end of the first week when it is clear that ventilation will have to be continued for some time. Tracheostomy is much more comfortable for the patient and allows normal eating and drinking.

Surgical emphysema

This is detected by the characteristic feeling of air in the tissues. Commonly, it is found in the immediate area of the fracture. Its importance lies in the fact that it must mean that the underlying lung has been damaged. Careful observation and a chest X-ray are therefore important to exclude a pneumothorax.

Sometimes, surgical emphysema will spread extensively from the fracture site to the scrotum and to the face and eyelids. This causes distress to the patient, relatives and the staff but is not in itself dangerous. However, such extensive emphysema must be due to a high pressure of gas in the tissues at the site of the fracture and consequently a pneumothorax is usually present, often of the tension type. An intercostal drain will treat the pneumothorax and lessen the progression of the emphysema. Distress to the patient can be minimized by careful explanation and by digital pressure on the eyelids. This disperses the emphysema and allows the patient to see.

Summary

Rib fractures alone are very painful and may lead to atelectasis of the underlying lung. Local anaesthesia is an effective method of treatment. Damage to underlying structures may cause a haemothorax or a pneumothorax, and either may progress to the dangerous tension stage. Intercostal drainage should be performed in all traumatic pneumo- or haemothoraces.

Flail chest leads to respiratory insufficiency, and is treated by mechanical ventilation for as long as it takes for the chest wall to heal and regain its normal rigidity.

Persisting controversies

- Ideal method of pain relief in chest wall injury.
- Desirability of suction on intercostal drains in traumatic pneumo- or haemothorax.
- Efficiency of external splinting of flail segments.

Damage to the lungs

In blunt chest injury, the lungs may be damaged by broken ribs or they may be contused as an indirect result of the deceleration induced by the accident (Fig. 4.2). This damage does not necessarily involve just the region of the trauma but may affect both lungs. Oedema and petechial haemorrhages follow, and the secretions of the lung into the alveoli and bronchial tree increase. Atelectasis and infection readily occur; there is also an impairment of oxygen uptake and, in severe cases, even the elimination of carbon dioxide.

All patients after blunt chest injuries have some degree of pulmonary dysfunction. At its most mild the patient may be unaffected by this but there will be a decrease in the ease of absorption of oxygen across the alveolar membrane detectable by estimation of the arterial blood gases. In its most severe manifestations, severe hypoxia, hypercarbia and very stiff lungs may occur in spite of mechanical ventilation.

Treatment of this complication is very difficult. Time is needed

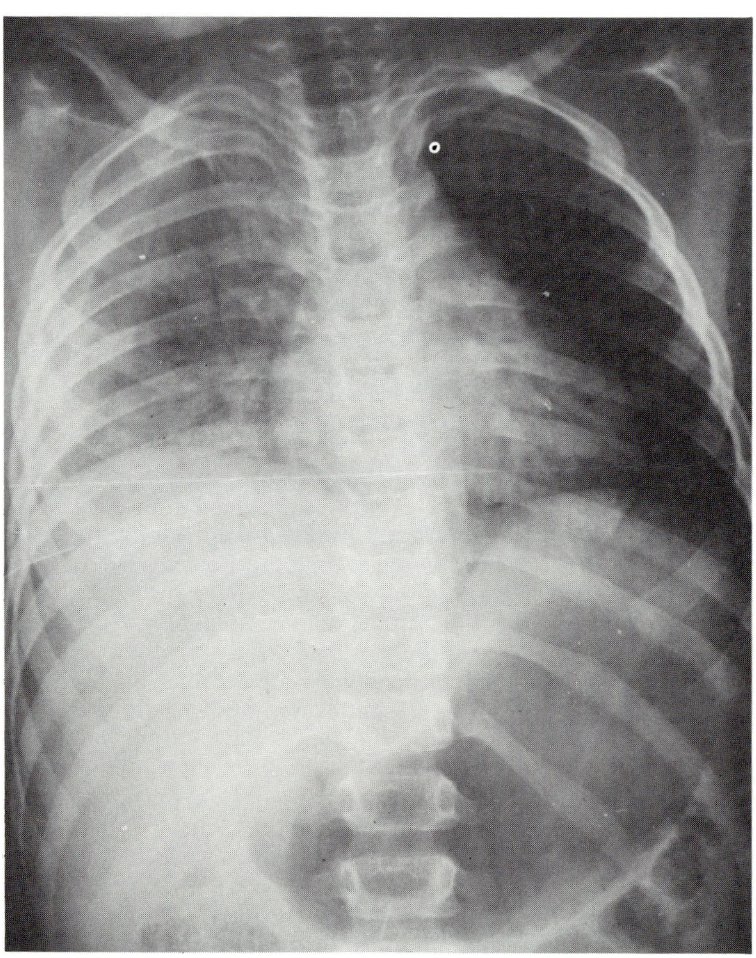

Figure 4.2
Chest X-ray showing a right haemothorax and extensive contusion of the right lung after a blunt chest injury. This patient subsequently died from severe respiratory failure caused by a superimposed pulmonary infection.

for the situation to resolve, but in the interim the patient may die of respiratory insufficiency, even if superadded infection can be avoided. Physiotherapy and skilled tracheobronchial toilet are useful in preventing infection.

Summary Contusion of the lungs occurs in blunt chest injury and time alone will lead to its resolution. Medical treatment consists of supporting the patient through the respiratory failure by appropriate means and by preventing infection.

Persisting controversy

- Do steroids help to resolve the contusion more quickly or is infection more likely to occur?

Damage to the mediastinum

Blunt trauma may damage the mediastinal organs (major airways, major vessels, heart or thoracic duct) by direct or indirect (deceleration) trauma.

Major airway damage Rupture of the trachea or major bronchi occurs as a result of deceleration. Airway injury should be suspected if:

1 Air is seen in the mediastinum on the X-ray.
2 Surgical emphysema of the neck is present.
3 A persisting and uncontrollable air leak prevents full expansion of the lung(s).

The slightest suspicion of damage to a major airway should lead to bronchoscopy. There are some dangers in discontinuing mechanical ventilation to use the rigid metallic bronchoscope, but the flexible fibre-optic bronchoscope may be inserted down the endotracheal tube while ventilation continues.

The trachea should be inspected from the glottis downwards and the major bronchi individually inspected. Sometimes a complete disruption of the entire wall may be seen but often there may be a localized haematoma. Such findings should lead to operative repair by thoractomy or, in the case of the upper trachea, by a cervical approach.

Major vessel damage Injury to the aorta and its major branches is the most common form of vascular injury in the mediastinum. Occasionally, damage to the inferior vena cava at its entry into the right atrium can occur. The injuries are produced by deceleration.

The damage may be a complete full thickness separation of the vessel and its surrounding tissues. In these cases, haemorrhage is rapid and fatal. More usually, the laceration spares the adventitia and the haemorrhage is slight for a period; only later does the patient exsanguinate. It is this group of patients which presents in hospital and which must be diagnosed in order to allow repair. Suspicion of major vascular injury should be ever present in blunt thoracic trauma. That suspicion should be doubled if there is any diminution of pulse in the limbs or neck or if there is any

Figure 4.3
(a) Chest X-ray of a patient admitted to a general ward after a blunt chest injury. He died suddenly when being moved for angiography. (b) Postmortem specimen of this patient's heart and aorta. Note transverse laceration in the descending aorta. (c) (opposite) Aortogram showing avulsion of the right innominate artery from the aorta.

(a)

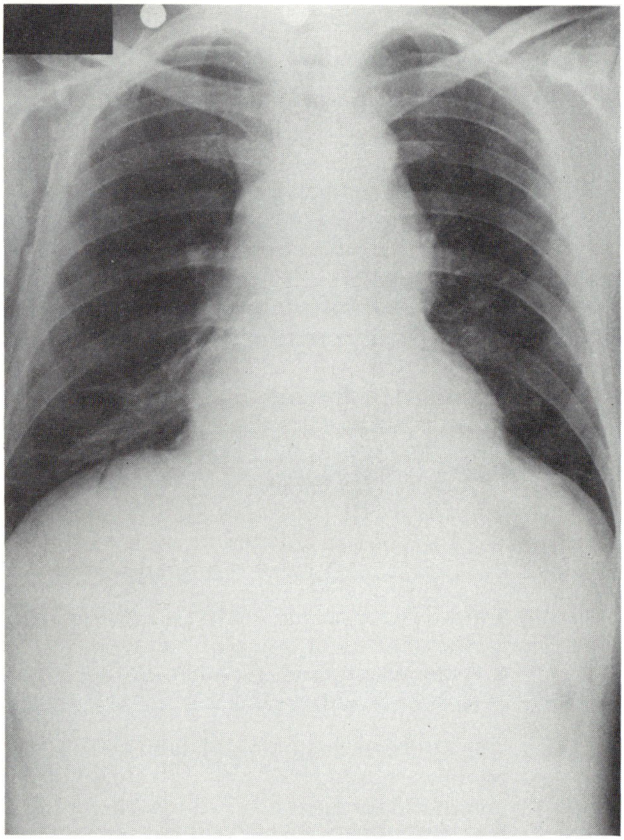

(b)

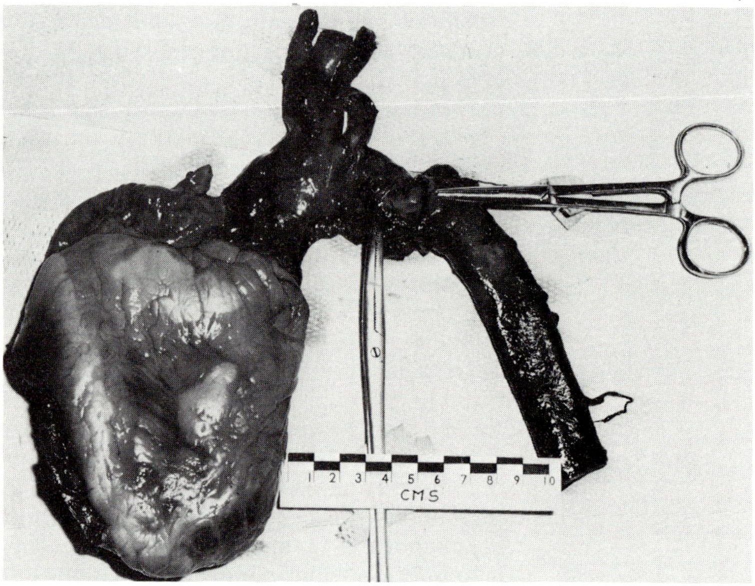

Figure 4.3 (c)

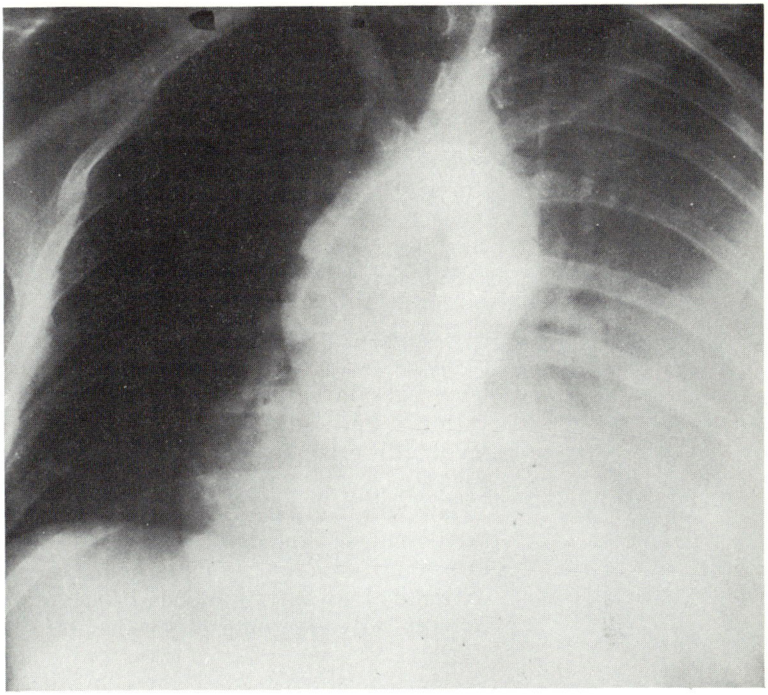

widening of the mediastinum on the chest X-ray. The chest X-ray taken in chest injuries is, of course, not a standard 6 ft postero-anterior film and thus 'widening' of the mediastinum may arise as a result of projection changes. Nevertheless, if major vessel injuries are to be diagnosed, all patients with a wide mediastinum on the chest X-ray should undergo aortography. To perform some unnecessary investigations is a small price to pay if these life-threatening but correctable injuries are not to be missed (Fig. 4.3). The most usual site of injury is the descending aorta, just below the origin of the left subclavian artery. Complete transverse transection of the vessel occurs and is amenable to repair, with or without left heart bypass, if diagnosed early. The origins of the innominate and carotid artery may be avulsed from the aorta and again repair should be undertaken. This group of patients frequently have fractures of the first rib and although the association is not complete, fracture of the first rib must arouse suspicion of vascular injury. Such lesions usually need full cardiopulmonary bypass to allow control of the vessels to effect repair.

Cardiac damage The heart, and in particular the right ventricle, lies immediately to the posterior of the sternum and it is not surprising that contusion of the myocardium may occur in blunt chest injury. Damage to the coronary arteries and to the valves has been recorded but is rare. Damage to the myocardium leads to an impairment of its contraction and a greater or lesser degree of cardiac failure. Occasionally, a haemopericardium may occur and cause tamponade.

Tamponade should be suspected if there is profound low output syndrome (see Chapter 5). If time permits, an echocardiogram will confirm the blood in the pericardium. Emergency left anterior thoracotomy should be performed immediately to release the blood. In the preparation for this, fatal compression of the heart may be avoided by needle aspiration of the pericardium.

Myocardial contusion causing a degree of cardiac failure is probably more common than has been thought. In severe cases, low output syndrome will occur and the right ventricle fails. In these cases, the indirect measurement of the left atrial pressure by a balloon catheter is essential if the management is to be rational. Serial 12-lead electrocardiographs will show changes of myocardial damage if scrutinized carefully by an expert interpreter.

The treatment of myocardial contusion is expectant. Once tamponade is excluded, myocardial support with inotropes or an afterload reducing agent is given for as long as necessary. In extreme cases, intra-aortic balloon counter-pulsation will theoretically salvage some otherwise fatally injured patients (see Chapter 5).

Damage to the thoracic duct

In those severe chest injuries which produce extension or severe distortion of the thoracic spine, the thoracic duct may rupture. This is a rare event and leads to chylothorax. This is diagnosed by examination of the fluid when the ensuing pleural effusion is aspirated. Most lesions of the thoracic duct will heal within a few days if adequate chest drain and lung expansion is achieved. However, if the drainage of chyle persists, the thoracic duct should be ligated since the patient will quickly run into severe nutritional problems.

Summary

Blunt chest injury may damage the lungs and mediastinal structures as well as the chest wall. Chest wall injuries are treated by pain relief and flail segments by mechanical ventilation. Some degree of pulmonary dysfunction always follows a blunt chest injury and, if severe, may be life threatening. Injury to the mediastinal structures is always life threatening and only suspicion and an aggressive policy of investigation will allow early diagnosis to be made, thus permitting early and effective treatment.

Persisting controversies

- Indications for aortography in suspected major vessel injury.
- The frequency and treatment of myocardial contusion.

Conclusion

Blunt chest trauma may damage every structure within the

chest. Although the injury may appear to be trivial, careful clinical and radiological assessment frequently repeated will uncover a group of patients with life-threatening complications. An aggressive policy of endoscopy and aortography is necessary to avoid missing highly treatable lesions. Respiratory failure of some degree is common in all cases of blunt chest injury and repeated assessments of pulmonary function are necessary to detect early deterioration.

Penetrating Chest Injuries

Penetrating wounds of the chest may cause damage to any intrathoracic organ; in addition, injury to the abdomen, spinal column and neck may also occur, depending on the direction of penetration. In civilian life the wound is not usually associated with extensive soft tissue damage around it, but in those injuries inflicted by military action there is always extensive damage which leads to further complications.

Indications for thoracotomy in penetrating chest injuries
Those countries with a high proportion of penetrating injuries have surgeons who are very experienced in the management of such cases and have the judgement as to when thoracotomy should be performed. Thus the standard teaching is that thoracotomy for penetrating injuries is only performed if an uncontrollable haemorrhage or air leak is present or *if there is the suspicion of damage to an intrathoracic viscus.* In those countries which are fortunate not to have a high proportion of penetrating injuries, there is usually insufficient experience to make a reliable judgement on this latter point. For this reason, we have practised a regimen of performing a small extendable thoracotomy on all patients with penetrating injuries of the chest. We have had no reason to regret this policy and on several occasions have found injury to intrathoracic organs which would have been undiagnosed until some major complication arose as a result.

A policy with regard to the management of penetrating injuries of the chest must be established and must take into account the continuing experience and skills of the medical staff looking after these patients. It is suggested that the standard teaching concerning thoracotomy does not apply to all units.

Persisting controversy

- The indications for thoracotomy in the patient with a penetrating chest injury.

Complications of penetrating chest injuries (Table 4.2)

Failure to diagnose the full extent of injury

Externally, the penetrating chest injury may appear to be trivial. A small puncture site over the chest wall in a patient who appears fit may lull the doctor into a state of false optimism. Often the

Table 4.2
Complications of penetrating chest injuries.

1 Failure to diagnose the full extent of injury
2 Damage to the lungs and bronchial tree
3 Damage to the heart and great vessels
4 Damage to the oesophagus
5 Damage to the diaphragm and intra-abdominal viscera

peripheral circumstances in which these incidents occur, such as crowd violence, drunkenness and abuse of other drugs, may give the doctor a wish to discharge the patient as rapidly as possible. A chest X-ray should always be performed if circumstances of clinical urgency permit. Even a small laceration of the chest should be explored under local anaesthesia in the Accident Department. Any suggestion that the amount of penetration is beyond the superficial muscles of the chest wall should make the patient be admitted for full assessment and observation.

On admission, an attempt must be made to gauge the type of weapon, its length and the angle of penetration. A downward direction to a stab wound may well injure and penetrate the apex of the dome of the diaphragm and injure the spleen or the liver. Similarly, a stab made in an upward direction may injure the structures passing over the apex of the lung, such as the brachial plexus or the subclavian vessels. However, it must be admitted that in most cases it is not possible to obtain an accurate history which will help resolve these worries.

In those units where there is great experience of penetrating injuries of the chest, sufficient expertise is accumulated to allow many patients with penetrating wounds to be observed and treated conservatively. In these units, only centrally placed injuries are submitted to thoracotomy. More lateral injuries are treated by the appropriate drainage of the pleural cavity and transfusion. Our policy, having relatively little experience of this sort of injury, has been to perform thoracotomy on every patient whose penetrating injury is thought to pass deeper than the muscles of the chest wall. A small lateral thoractomy is not upsetting to the patient and permits the surgeon to inspect all of the structures in that hemithorax. Some patients have had fruitless explorations. Others have had surprising findings. One had an amputation of the tip of the left atrial appendix from a lateral stab wound with a kitchen knife. No bleeding was seen at the time because of clotting around the cardiac injury. Another had penetration of the right dome of the diaphragm and a laceration of the liver. Yet another had had a chest drain inserted in the left chest for a haemothorax following a stab injury. On arrival at our hospital, thoracotomy revealed that the drain had transfixed the descending aorta. We feel, therefore, that our policy of performing open exploration of all penetrating chest injuries is justified but respect those with larger experience whose judgement is less fallible.

Summary. In those units with a limited experience of penetrating chest injuries, exploratory thoracotomy will reduce the chance of missing severe visceral injury and relieve the surgeon of much anxiety.

Damage to the lungs and bronchial tree

Damage to these structures, if severe, will lead to a haemopneumothorax on admission and this may be under tension. If so, the patient may be so ill that there is no time to perform a chest X-ray. The principle needs to be repeated: if the mediastinum, as judged by the position of the trachea, is grossly deviated in a moribund patient, a chest drain should be inserted into the hemithorax away from which the mediastinum has shifted. At the same time, massive transfusion of blood or plasma will be needed to restore circulating blood volume.

When the drain is inserted and the lung expands, the bleeding usually ceases fairly rapidly. If a repeat chest X-ray shows full expansion and the bleeding has stopped, the surgeon of great experience may choose to observe the patient. For the reasons stated above, we would perform a thoracotomy.

If the lung does not expand, either because of uncontrollable bleeding or air leak or there is radiological evidence of clotted blood within the haemothorax, there is universal agreement that a full thoracotomy should be performed as soon as the patient's condition permits.

At operation, pleural clot is removed and the lung carefully inspected. Lacerations of the pulmonary parenchyma are oversewn with buttressed sutures and the major pulmonary vessels at the hilum inspected. The chest wall, diaphragm and mediastinum are carefully scrutinized and, in particular, the pericardium opened through a small incision to exclude blood. The chest is then closed with two drains – one apical and one basal – and any devitalized tissues in the chest wound excised. Tetanus prophylaxis and an antibiotic are given.

After operation, some degree of respiratory dysfunction will occur because of the ecchymosis and contusion of the lung surrounding the injury. Given time, adequate analgesia and physiotherapy, spontaneous resolution will occur.

Lacerations of the trachea and bronchus are suggested by surgical emphysema in the mediastinum or neck and are confirmed by endoscopy. When thoracotomy is performed, direct repair of the laceration is performed using multiple interrupted non-absorbable sutures. Adequate drainage of the surrounding tissues is essential.

Damage to the heart and great vessels

Most patients with penetrating wounds of the heart or great vessels will arrive moribund. Usually, this is due to cardiac tamponade rather than blood loss, although the latter is also present. Any penetrating injury over the front of the chest and within the midclavicular lines is likely to have inflicted cardiac injury.

Emergency endotracheal intubation and blood transfusion are set up and some means of relieving the cardiac compression must then be performed. Needle aspiration of the pericardium will give temporary relief but is made unreliable by the inherent difficulties of the procedure. Probably the most reliable way of decompressing the pericardium in a moribund patient is to perform a small anterior thoracotomy, along the line of the left fifth rib, just below the left nipple. The tense, bulging pericardium is then opened anteriorly to the left phrenic nerve and the blood allowed to gush out. This procedure must often be carried out in the Accident Department and a set of instruments for this purpose should be available. When the tamponade is relieved, there remains the less urgent problem of haemorrhage. This can be resolved in a less frenetic manner by taking the patient to an operating theatre where the thoracotomy can be extended and the wounds identified and repaired.

When should the emergency evacuation of tamponade not be performed? Obviously, not when a patient is other than moribund. Less obviously, some units have reported the results of relieving tamponade in patients who arrive at the hospital clinically dead with dilated pupils and no heart action. Although many of these patients remain dead, a surprisingly large minority survive the experience and leave hospital. Emergency room thoracotomy is therefore justified on all patients who arrive moribund with penetrating injuries to the heart or great vessels. In the operating theatre, full resuscitation and thoracotomy are performed. Most penetrating wounds of the heart and great vessels can be repaired without the use of cardiopulmonary bypass.

Damage to the oesophagus

A deeply penetrating wound may lacerate this most inaccessible structure. A small laceration may lead to mediastinitis only, but most will lead to a hydrothorax on the side of the injury. Aspiration of the fluid will lead to diagnosis and this will be confirmed by a contrast study in the radiological department.

If the diagnosis is made within four hours of the injury, primary repair may be possible; otherwise, the area of the injury should be drained and a gastrostomy performed. The patient should not be allowed oral food or drink until radiological confirmation of healing is obtained. A temporary cervical oesophagostomy may ensure more adequate defunctioning of the injured area.

Damage to the diaphragm and intra-abdominal viscera

The shape of the diaphragm leads to the possibility that any penetrating wound of the thorax will penetrate the diaphragm and lead to intra-abdominal injury (Fig. 4.4). Clearly, the lower the wound, the stronger the possibility. The maximal height of the domes of the diaphragm should be assumed to be at the level of the nipples in males and the fifth intercostal space in females. Consequently, part of the clinical assessment of the patient with a penetrating chest injury is to repeatedly examine the abdomen.

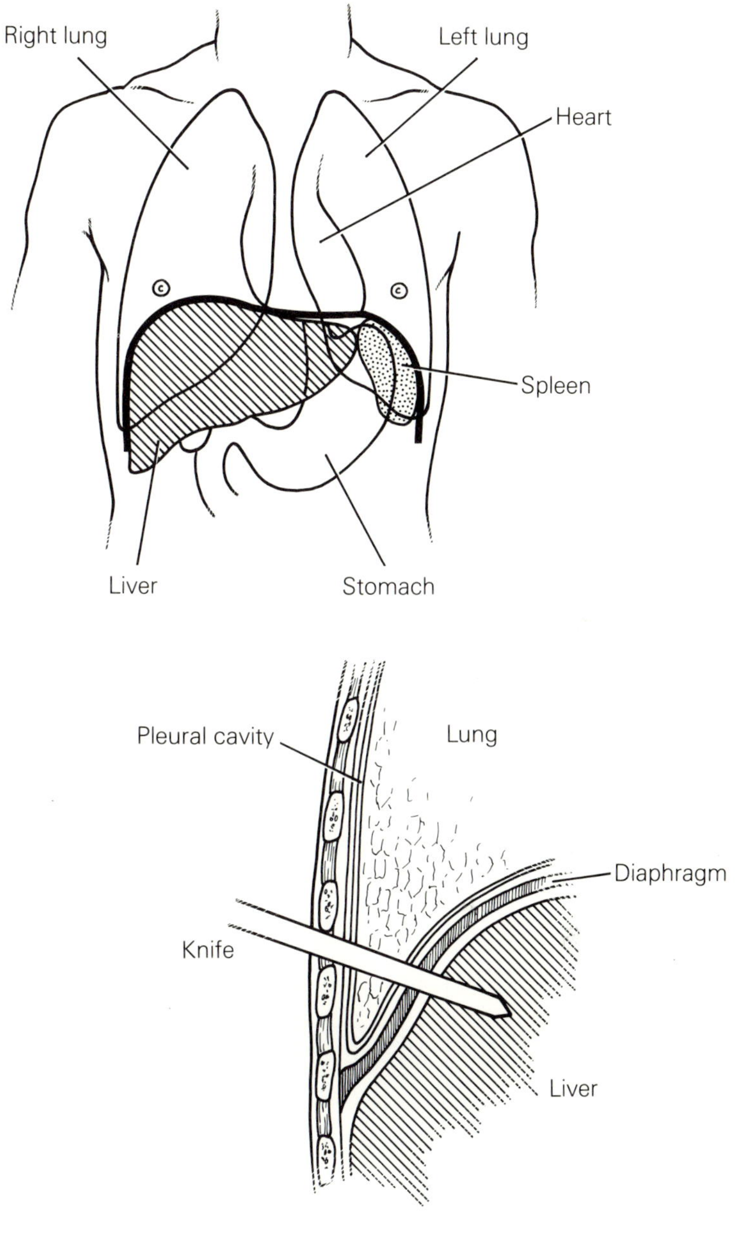

Figure 4.4
Anatomy of the diaphragm showing how a chest wound may involve the intra-abdominal viscera.

Any evidence of tenderness or rigidity should raise this possibility. Obviously, if a policy of thoracotomy for penetrating wounds is adopted, these injuries will be detected at an early stage. Intra-abdominal injuries are managed in the conventional way. The laceration of the diaphragm is repaired with multiple thick unabsorbable sutures.

Summary

Penetrating wounds of the chest are uncommon in many parts of the world. The wounds inflicted in civilian life are not usually accompanied by much soft tissue damage, whereas those arising from military conflict may have extensive damage needing treatment in its own right. Any intrathoracic organ may be damaged by a penetrating wound. Even in patients who appear fit, it is suggested that an aggressive policy of thoracotomy should be followed in order to prevent avoidable complications. Injuries to the heart and great vessels are often fatal and an aggressive policy of tamponade relief should be practised. Any penetrating wound of the chest may cause intra-abdominal injury.

Persisting controversies

- Indications for thoracotomy in penetrating chest injuries.
- Usefulness of pericardial aspiration in the injuries of the heart.
- The use of blood saving systems in the management of massive haemorrhage.

Further reading

Grover, F.L., Ellestad, C., Arom, K.V., Root, H.D., Cruz, A.B. & Trinkle, J.K. (1979) Diagnosis and management of major tracheo-bronchial injuries. *Ann. Thorac. Surg.*, *28*, 378.

Kirsh, M.M. & Sloan, H. (ed.) (1977) *Blunt Chest Trauma; General Principles of Management.* Boston: Little, Brown and Company.

Symbas, P.N. (1972) *Traumatic Injuries to the Heart and Great Vessels.* Springfield, Illinois: Charles C. Thomas.

5 Complications of Cardiac Surgery

The function of the heart is to produce an adequate flow of blood to all the tissues of the body. This pump function is complex in its mechanisms and control but compared with other organs such as the liver and kidney is relatively simple physiologically. Cardiac surgical operations which improve the mechanical efficiency of the heart should have an immediately beneficial effect to both the heart as an organ and the patient as a whole. This feature distinguishes cardiac surgery from nearly all other surgery and permits operations to be performed on gravely ill patients with a good prospect of relief. In common with other surgical operations, however, cure is only rarely achieved. Most operations are palliative; because the relief of the condition may last for years or even decades this does not alter the essentially palliative nature of most cardiac surgery.

The early years of cardiac surgery were judged according to the mortality of the operations and their immediate morbidity. As the risks of surgery became lower, a further criterion, that of long-term function recovery, was added. Many routine cardiac operations now have an immediate hospital mortality of under 3% and such a low figure is too insensitive to allow a proper judgement of the value of any particular procedure to be made. The nature and degree of the long-term functional recovery is much more sensitive as an index of the value of an operation. Paradoxically, since surgeons have paid attention to this feature and sought ways of improving long-term function, the immediate mortality of the operations has fallen as a direct result.

In this chapter, the avoidance and management of complications of cardiac surgery will deal with the immediate and long-term complications which may prevent the patient returning to a normal life.

The concern of cardiac surgeons to reduce mortality and morbidity and to improve long-term function is not a simple issue. A very low hospital mortality for any procedure can be achieved by denying the benefit of the operation to those individuals who are at higher risk. Those surgeons who believe that the risk of surgery is irrelevant, if it is less than the risk of not operating, are bound to have higher global mortality and morbidity figures and yet these surgeons will extend the benefits of cardiac surgery to a much wider group of patients. The decision about whether a patient is inoperable is complex and is influenced not only by the hard facts of surgical and non-surgical risk but also by the philosophy of both the surgeon and the patient. In addition, the strengths and experience of the particular surgical team have to be considered. Some units, for instance, have surgeons and supporting staff who are particularly expert and experienced in certain conditions. It would be foolish for others not to consider such factors when making surgical decisions.

In summary, cardiac surgical operations are nearly always palliative but tend to offer immediate improvement of function. Complications of cardiac surgery lead not only to increased mortality and morbidity but more importantly to an impairment of function in the years that follow surgery. Crude mortality figures may be very misleading and depend largely on case selection.

Cardiac operations are of two types, the 'closed' and the 'open'. In 'closed' cardiac operations, the procedure is performed on a heart which is supporting the circulation. Such procedures are inevitably somewhat limited in their scope and simple in nature, and are often performed 'blindly', i.e. not under direct vision. Closed mitral valvotomy is an example of a closed operation. 'Open' operations are performed on a heart which is not supporting the circulation. While the operation is being done, the rest of the body has to have its metabolic needs met. This may be achieved either by cardiopulmonary bypass, as described separately (see Chapter 6), or by reduction of the body's metabolism by hypothermia. Open operations permit more complex repairs to be performed under direct vision. Replacement of a cardiac valve is always performed under open conditions. Operations on the coronary arteries are performed on a non-beating heart but, although described as such, are not truly open operations in that there is no opening into a cardiac chamber during the procedure.

Myocardial function. Cardiac operations, whether performed for congenital defects or upon the valves or coronary arteries, are rarely concerned principally with the myocardium. The function of the myocardium, however, is clearly important both before and after the operation. If in spite of adequate correction of the surgical lesion damage to the myocardium occurs in the perioperative period, clearly the pumping function of the heart will be diminished. The myocardial damage may be temporary or permanent depending on its cause. If severe, the damage may kill the patient during or immediately after the operation. Less severe degrees of damage may permit a patient to survive but not allow a full functional recovery. In the last ten years, the cardinal importance of myocardial function has been appreciated. Some cardiac lesions obviously cause myocardial damage. The left ventricular muscle is likely to be damaged in patients with chronic aortic or mitral valve disease. Correction of the haemodynamic problem will cause an immediate improvement in heart function, provided that no further damage occurs to the myocardium during the course of that correction. Sometimes such damage may be inevitable but very often the damage occurs because of a lack of awareness of the physiological needs of the myocardium. These needs and the ways in which they can be met are grouped together and called 'myocardial protection'. Adequate myocardial protection will ensure adequate cardiac function after the operation. It is justifiable in discussing the complications of cardiac surgery to deal with myocardial protection in some detail as the major preventive measure available.

In summary, whatever type of operation is performed, correction of the haemodynamic abnormality should lead to an immediate improvement in cardiac function. If the heart is less competent after an operation, either the correction has not been perfect or myocardial damage has occurred. Myocardial damage should be regarded as an avoidable complication of cardiac surgery and efforts made to minimize it both during the operation and in the perioperative period.

Myocardial Preservation

Physiology of the myocardium

The heart muscle derives its contractile power from aerobic metabolism. A very limited capacity for anaerobic metabolism exists and for practical purposes may be ignored. The oxygen necessary for aerobic metabolism is delivered in arterial blood flowing through the coronary arteries into the vascular bed of the myocardium. The tissue demand for oxygen will be determined by the work done by the myocardium. Normally, there will be equilibrium between the availability of oxygen and the demand for oxygen from the myocardium. If the demand exceeds the availability, sooner or later damage to the energy producing systems in the myocardial cells will occur.

Most of the cardiac work is performed by the left ventricle (LV). The major determinant of cardiac oxygen consumption is therefore left ventricular work. Clearly, the higher the pressure generated by the LV, and the longer that pressure is sustained, the more oxygen will be used. Thus oxygen demand will be related to the area under the left ventricular pressure tracing (Fig. 5.1). This area is called the 'systolic tension time index' (STTI) and is an index of oxygen consumption by the left ventricle. Oxygen availability will be determined largely by the blood flow through the coronary circulation, assuming adequate levels of oxygenated haemoglobin. Coronary arterial flow is phasic and within the inner myocardium, particularly, occurs during diastole only. Thus the flow to the muscle is dependent upon the diastolic blood pressure and the length of diastole. In Fig. 5.1, the hatched area between the diastolic aortic tracing and the left ventricular diastolic pressure represents the diastolic pressure time index (DPTI) and thus oxygen availability.

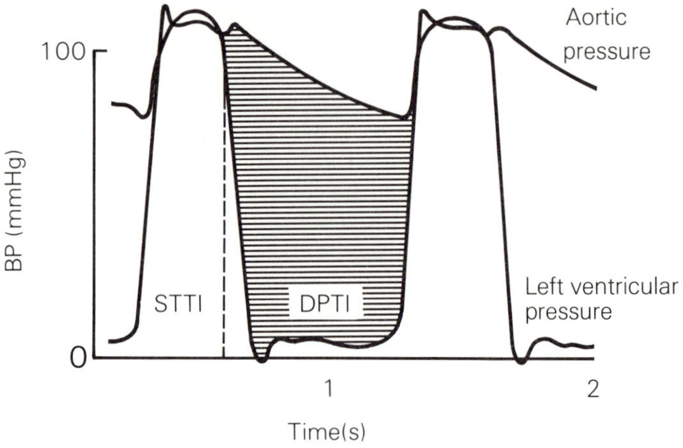

Figure 5.1 Pressures within the aorta and left ventricle during the cardiac cycle. STTI=systolic tension time index, DPTI=diastolic pressure time index.

Experimental studies in both animals and humans have shown that normally STTI and DPTI are equal (i.e. DPTI/STTI = 1). By various manipulations of the intracardiac and aortic pressures, and of the heart rate, investigators have altered the STTI and DPTI in experimental animals. Once the DPTI/STTI ratio becomes 0.5 or less, myocardial damage leading to necrosis will occur within the inner myocardium in normal animals. In animals with hypertrophied ventricles or coronary arterial lesions, the DPTI/STTI ratio has to be reduced only a little below 1 to cause damage.

What are the clinical implications of this elegant work? First, a reservation. The experimental observations were carried out with intracavity transducers and extremely accurate recording equipment. It is not normally possible to use such equipment clinically and therefore the pressure measurements and timing do not permit a precise mathematical analysis of STTI and DPTI at the bedside. Most patients with heart disease at least have the possibility of coronary arterial disease which will further limit oxygen availability to the myocardium.

However, despite this reservation the concept that STTI and DPTI should be equal does suggest certain strategies which may be employed to avoid myocardial damage in the pre- and postoperative period.

1 Tachycardia should be avoided. Pulse rates of more than 120/min reduce the period of diastole and therefore coronary filling. The cause of the tachycardia should be sought and treated.
2 The arterial blood pressure should not be allowed to rise above about 140 mmHg systolic.
3 The left ventricular end diastolic pressure should not be allowed to rise above 15 mmHg.

In practice, these points are determined and controlled by

accurate and continuous measurements of the arterial blood pressure, the pulse rate and perhaps the left atrial or pulmonary artery pressure. Since the period of risk for the surgical patient begins long before the operation, cannulation of the various vessels in order to measure the pressure and electrocardiograph recording is started *before* the induction of anaesthesia. Cannulation under local anaesthesia will not upset the suitably premedicated adult patient, but children are lightly anaesthetized first.

After the operation, monitoring of the ECG and arterial pressures is continued and adjusted accordingly.

Summary The oxygen requirement and oxygen availability of the myocardium must be closely matched or damage will occur. The systolic tension time index (STTI) and the diastolic tension time index (DPTI) provide a means of understanding the magnitude of these factors.

Myocardial preservation during the operation

Cardiopulmonary bypass does not provide the best conditions for delivery of oxygen to the myocardium. The flow is non-pulsatile and at a variable pressure. In addition, there is always the possibility of microemboli causing small vessel obstruction. These factors compound the problems of perfusing a hypertrophied myocardium and possible coronary disease further complicates the picture.

In addition, the surgeon finds it very difficult to operate on a beating heart and there is always the possibility of a beating heart causing arterial air embolism. Ventricular fibrillation can be induced electrically and gives much improved operating conditions. However, the oxygen consumption of fibrillating myocardium is three to four times that of normally contracting muscle and tissue hypoxia is very easily caused. Consequently during cardiopulmonary bypass it is very difficult to supply the oxygen requirements of the heart.

Most surgeons have now abandoned the attempt to supply the myocardium with sufficient oxygen and rely instead on reducing the requirements to as low as possible so that the needs are more easily met. The usual way at present to achieve this is to paralyse the heart with a high (20–30 mmol/l) potassium solution. This preserves intracellular energy stores. The metabolism of the myocardium is then reduced by cooling with 4 °C solutions applied via the coronary arteries and externally via the pericardium. Hypothermic hyperkalaemic solutions achieving this paralysis are called 'cardioplegic' solutions.

The cardioplegic solution is run through the coronary arteries under pressure after clamping the ascending aorta. Immediate asystole is produced and maintained until the coronary circulation is restarted by removing the aortic clamp. Properly used, hypothermic hyperkalaemic cardioplegia permits ideal operating conditions and produces a better return of ventricular function after bypass than any other form of intraoperative myocardial protection.

Hypothermic cardioplegic arrest of the heart during cardiopulmonary bypass is not universally used. Many simple lesions may be corrected during a short period – say up to 20 minutes – of aortic cross-clamping. Many surgeons perform coronary artery operations on the fibrillating heart with aortic cross-clamping, with results that are identical to those obtained with cardioplegia. Most surgeons use cardioplegia as their preferred method of myocardial preservation during valve replacement surgery. At the time of writing, cardioplegia is very popular and widely used but other methods of myocardial preservation are used.

The patient who requires inotropic support to treat low output syndrome after cardiac surgery (see below) has sustained myocardial damage. Such damage may be unavoidable in this particular operation but otherwise should be regarded as an avoidable hazard which has the potential to cause mortality, morbidity and an impaired functional recovery. Attention to the principles outlined above will greatly reduce the incidence of myocardial damage with benefit to the patient.

Finally, the need for perioperative myocardial preservation is not confined to cardiac surgical patients. The factors governing myocardial oxygen demand and availability are important to *any* patient undergoing surgery. Haemorrhage and other physiological disturbances can even affect patients with normal hearts and it is not uncommon for patients with diseased hearts to present as abdominal surgical emergencies or to suffer trauma. The skill with which the surgical team looks after such patients will determine the risk of cardiac damage occurring and therefore the chances of the patients surviving the illness.

Summary During operation, damage to the myocardium will follow if oxygen demand and availability are not identical. Damage may be avoided by supplying adequate oxygen or by reducing the demand by the use of hypothermic hyperkalaemic cardioplegia. Difficulties of adequate supply may be exacerbated by ventricular hypertrophy, coronary arterial disease and by the artificial nature of cardiopulmonary bypass. For these reasons, and for technical ease, many surgeons prefer to use cardioplegia.

Low Cardiac Output Syndrome (Shock)

Low cardiac output syndrome is defined as the state in which the cardiac output is insufficient to support the metabolic needs of the body tissues. The cardinal derangement is therefore in cardiac function and it is appropriate to deal with the syndrome in a comprehensive manner in this volume. However, low output syndrome (LOS) is far from being exclusive to cardiac surgery, although it is certainly common. LOS may occur in any branch of surgery and full discussion, with perhaps some overlap with other volumes in this series, is justified because of the frequency of the syndrome and the widespread medical and surgical misconceptions surrounding it.

The term 'shock' was previously used to describe LOS but was very difficult to define. Every specialty had its own special brand of shock and the treatments varied accordingly. The only common factor between the varieties of shock was a very high mortality and a poor understanding of the physiological derangements caused by it. In the late 1950s and 1960s, however, the experience gained on the battlefield led to well-designed studies which cast light on the aetiology and treatment of shock. However, the term 'shock' had become so abused and imprecise by this stage that a more accurate term had to be found, even if a degree of verbal pomposity was introduced.

Diagnosis of LOS

The essential feature of LOS is a low cardiac output. The normal metabolic requirements of the body tissues demand a certain level of perfusion and once perfusion falls below that level, physiological derangement will occur and ultimately tissue damage. Clearly, normal cardiac output will depend on the size of the body tissue mass. Physiologically, the body tissue mass is most closely related to body surface area which is calculated by the height and weight by standard nomograms. The average adult male, for instance, has a body surface area of approximately 1.8 m^2 and the adult female approximately 1.5 m^2. The ideal cardiac output at rest is 3.2 $l/min \cdot m^{-2}$ body surface area (expressed as the 'cardiac index' of 3.2). Thus the average male needs a cardiac output at rest of $3.2 \times 1.8 = 5.7$ l/min. Once the cardiac index falls below 2.2, signs of impaired tissue perfusion occur and LOS is present.

The diagnosis of LOS is ideally made by measuring cardiac output and finding the cardiac index below 2.2. In practice, measurement of cardiac output has been difficult until recently and not applicable to the urgent clinical situation of LOS. Measurement of cardiac output is now made more widely available and easier by thermodilution techniques, but it is certainly not used for the majority of patients with LOS because of its expense and the need to insert a catheter into the right heart chambers.

Instead, the clinical diagnosis of LOS is made by demonstrating that the tissues of the body are failing to function properly as a result of impaired perfusion. When malfunction of many body tissues occurs from this cause, clearly the underlying reason must be a low cardiac output.

Main signs of LOS (see Fig. 5.4)

1 Poor urinary output (less than 0.5 ml/kg body weight$\cdot h^{-1}$).
2 Impaired skin perfusion leading to low temperature.

3 Low arterial blood pressure (less than 70 mmHg).
4 Progressive metabolic acidosis.

Some amplification of the above four points is needed in order to make some physiological sense.

Urinary output. The kidneys have a function which is easily and rapidly measured by inserting a catheter into the bladder. Clearly, the production of urine will depend on renal perfusion. More importantly, if renal perfusion is adequate the perfusion of the other viscera is also adequate and thus urinary flow is a good guide to visceral perfusion in general. The flow of urine will vary very quickly with changes in cardiac output.

Skin perfusion. Impaired cardiac output leads to skin vasoconstriction and a lowered temperature. This is a most useful physical sign and ideally should be continually measured electronically so that trends may be recorded accurately. However, the surgeon's hand will detect a cold foot easily enough to be reliable in the first instance.

Arterial pressure. The blood pressure may or may not vary with changes in cardiac output because there will be compensating changes in the peripheral resistance of the vascular system. Such a compensating system has a clear biological advantage in that the brain is perfused adequately at the expense of the other tissues of the body. However, it does make the level of the arterial pressure unhelpful in assessing cardiac output. Nevertheless, there are two tissues, the brain and the myocardium, which rely on pressure for their perfusion and thus the level of the blood pressure is important (but less so than skin temperature and urinary output and even then only within wide limits). In practice, this means that the patient with a blood pressure of 120/80, cold skin and no urinary output is a cause for considerable concern. Another patient with a blood pressure of 80/60, warm skin and an excellent urinary output is in no danger.

Metabolic acidosis. Progressive metabolic acidosis occurs late in LOS as a result of increasing skeletal muscle anaerobic metabolism. It is not very helpful in the early diagnosis of LOS but important in its effects.

Summary

The diagnosis of low cardiac output syndrome (LOS) should be made on the effects of poor tissue perfusion. Urine output is the most useful observation, followed by skin temperature. Blood pressure is much less important and then only within wide limits. Direct measurement of the cardiac output is the ideal way to diagnose the syndrome but although increasingly used remains too expensive and invasive to allow its universal application. The term 'shock' with its inevitable association of low blood pressure should be abandoned.

Persisting controversies

- The indications and place of direct measurement of the cardiac output in the management of LOS.
- The expanding indications for indirect left atrial pressure measurement.

Detection of the cause of LOS

The heart may fail to produce an adequate output for two reasons only. Either it is failing as a pump (cardiogenic LOS) or it is failing to be filled properly by the venous return (hypovolaemic LOS). There are many reasons why either derangement should occur (these are shown in the flow diagram on page 85).

Failure of the heart as a pump is called 'cardiogenic' failure. Insufficient filling of the heart is due to an inadequate volume of circulating blood which is termed 'hypovolaemia'. The important first step in diagnosing the cause of LOS is to determine whether cardiogenic or hypovolaemic factors are operating. The distinction is made by measuring the central venous pressure (CVP), i.e. the pressure within the right atrium or intrathoracic great veins. There is no clinical method of measuring this pressure and it is necessary to insert a catheter into the right atrium via an arm or neck vein (Fig. 5.2). The catheter is then attached to a conventional intravenous giving set and used mostly as a drip. However, a side-arm will allow measurement of the central venous pressure in terms of the height of a column of fluid within the side-arm (Fig. 5.3).

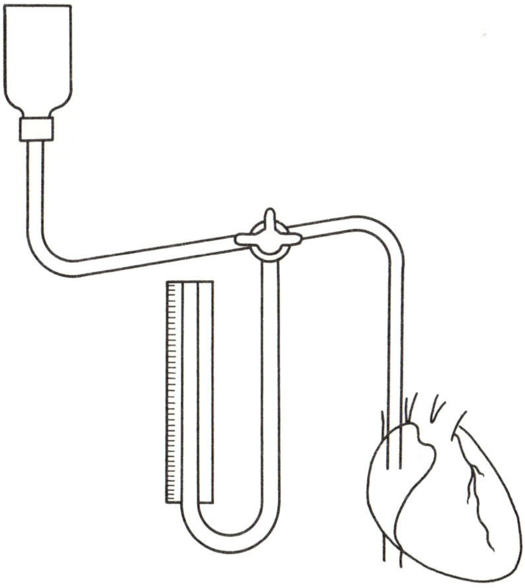

Figure 5.2
Measurement of right atrial pressure.

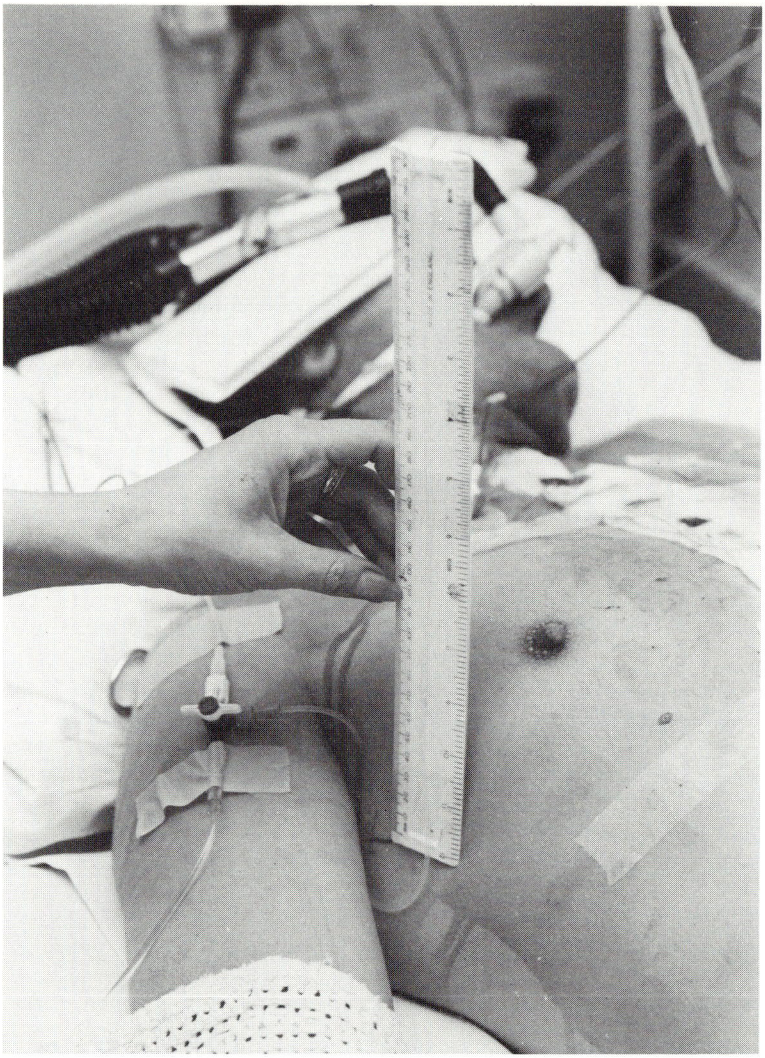

Figure 5.3
Measurement of central venous pressure. The patient has an internal jugular line in position.

Measurement of the central venous pressure (CVP) is essential to distinguish between cardiogenic and hypovolaemic LOS. If the CVP is below 5 mmHg, hypovolaemia is certainly present. Similarly, if the CVP is 20 mmHg or more, the cause for the LOS is cardiogenic. Like any other observation, however, the CVP, although highly reliable, has deficits and should not be accepted without some cautions. One drawback of CVP measurement is that it measures pressures in the right heart only and the assumption is made that the normal equality between right and left atrial pressures is retained. This may be wrong at times and most hearts which fail do so in consequence of left ventricular dysfunction. In these circumstances, the left atrial pressure may be much higher than the right. Another problem of CVP measurement is that the filling pressures of the heart may be maintained in hypovolaemia by a variable degree of venospasm. Thus the CVP may be maintained near normal by constriction of the veins even in the presence of significant hypovolaemia.

The attending surgeon needs to be aware of these drawbacks to CVP measurement. Should the possibility of left heart failure be strong, an indirect measurement of left atrial pressure may be made either by a pulmonary wedge pressure or by measurement of the diastolic pressure in the pulmonary artery, both of which give a reliable indication of left atrial pressure. Direct measurement of left atrial pressure is only possible by inserting a catheter at the time of operation and this is frequently done in high-risk cardiac cases.

The effect of venopasm may be assessed by the rapid infusion of a small volume – say 200 ml – of fluid to the patient. Should the CVP remain unchanged, or perhaps rise a little, there is a strong possibility of venospasm masking a significant degree of hypovolaemia.

The fact that CVP measurement has its drawbacks does not diminish its value in the diagnosis of the cause of LOS. Certainly, not to use CVP measurement at all because of its known drawbacks is illogical and will cause more problems than if it is used in a manner which appreciates its limitations.

Summary

Measurement of CVP will distinguish between most cases of hypovolaemic and cardiogenic LOS. CVP measurement is not infallible, however, and needs to be interpreted carefully with the possibility of left heart failure and venospasm. Nevertheless, it remains a very useful measurement without which rational management of LOS becomes very difficult. In the practice of cardiac surgery, indirect or direct measurement of left atrial pressure will frequently be needed because of left ventricular disease.

Persisting controversy

- Indications for and limitations of CVP measurement.

Treatment of hypovolaemic LOS (see flow diagram on page 85)
First, the blood volume is restored by infusion of whatever seems appropriate. Second, the lesion which has led to hypovolaemia should be corrected. In haemorrhage, for instance, bleeding should be controlled at the same time if possible. In patients who are suffering from LOS due to water and salt depletion, the cause should be sought for and remedied. Once the CVP has been restored to normal, the indirect indices of tissue perfusion and cardiac output are reassessed. If they have resolved, it is likely that the cause of the LOS was simply hypovolaemia and that it has been corrected. However, the cause is often not simple and

LOS remains. The reversal of hypovolaemia is the first step in the treatment of such complicated cases.

During this phase, large quantities of fluid may have to be infused. If blood is used, it should be warmed to physiological levels and should be passed through a microfilter to remove microemboli which cause pulmonary damage and dysfunction.

Treatment of cardiogenic LOS (see flow diagram opposite)
If LOS is present with a normal or raised CVP, or if LOS persists after correction of a low CVP, the cause is probably cardiogenic, bearing in mind the reservations already expressed about CVP measurement.

The next crucial step is to decide if the cardiac dysfunction is being caused by a removable mechanical problem. Such problems as tamponade or a thrombosed valvular prosthesis clearly need surgical solutions, whereas problems of myocardial function are unlikely to have a simple solution. Although crucial as a step, the distinction may not always be simple to make. To detect a malfunctioning cardiac valve may need cardiac catheterization, for instance, and even then the answer may be unclear. The diagnosis of cardiac tamponade is particularly difficult and the classic signs of a falling cardiac output with a rising CVP may be very late. Certainly, in cases where a strong possibility of tamponade exists and where other treatments have not been successful, exploratory operation is justified in order to exclude the condition. Should tamponade be found, it should of course be remedied. If tamponade is not found, at least the element of doubt has been removed at very little cost to the patient. Such operations must involve opening the whole wound and chest wall. Limited operations performed via a small incision are of as little value as non-invasive tests such as echocardiography.

Cardiac tamponade

Cardiac tamponade may be suspected after cardiac surgery if there is or has been excessive bleeding from the chest drains or an intermittent pattern of drainage is seen. The LOS which occurs tends to be very unresponsive to other treatments and to be associated with an unremitting tachycardia. The older textbooks of cardiac surgery emphasized the 'pulseless' nature of tamponade, meaning that the pulse volume was so low as to prevent easy palpation of even quite major peripheral arteries such as the brachials or femorals.

The sound physiological practice of infusing blood according to the CVP clouds the diagnosis of cardiac tamponade because the infusion is stopped as the CVP begins to rise. In difficult cases where tamponade is suspected, a bolus infusion of say 200 ml of blood will cause a dramatic rise in CVP and a deterioration of the cardiac output.

Having decided that tamponade and mechanical factors are not present, the treatment of cardiogenic LOS becomes more difficult because the problem is usually myocardial, and in order

Suggested plan of treatment of low output syndrome (LOS)

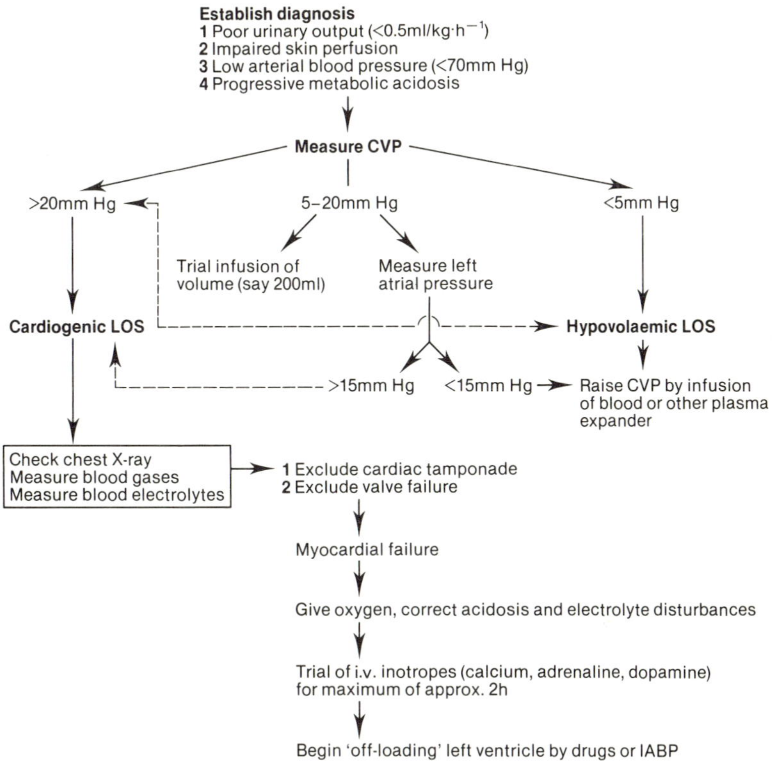

to reverse the low cardiac output the power of the myocardium has to be increased. This increased contraction will, of course, demand more oxygen via the coronary circulation and unless this can be provided increased work will lead to increasing myocardial damage. This problem has already been described above (page 75).

Drugs As described in the flow diagram (see above), the first step is to correct abnormally slow rates either by pacing or some chronotropic drug such as isoprenaline. Next, metabolic abnormalities such as electrolyte or acid–base disturbances or arterial hypoxia should be corrected by whatever means is appropriate. If LOS is still present, drug therapy is needed. Two broad types of drugs are used in myocardial failure leading to LOS. First are the inotropic drugs, such as adrenaline and dopamine, which increase the force of contraction of the heart and often also its rate. Second, the contractile state of the left ventricle and the cardiac output may be increased by manipulation of the 'afterload' of the left ventricle.

Inotropic drugs undoubtedly increase the cardiac output by making the myocardium contract more strongly. This increase in contraction has to be paid for by an increased oxygen *consumption* and therefore the oxygen *demand* of the heart increases. Unfortunately, an inadequate supply of oxygen is often the fundamental disturbance causing the LOS in the first place. Inotropic drugs may therefore increase myocardial damage if used unwisely. If they are used, the hope is held that the increase of cardiac output will cause a parallel increase in coronary flow and oxygen availability.

In practice, this means that a weak solution of adrenaline (4 mg in 500 ml isotonic saline), dopamine (800 mg in 500 ml isotonic saline) or isoprenaline (2 mg in 500 ml isotonic saline) is given at a controlled rate intravenously. For reasons already stated, tachycardia of more than 110/minute should be avoided. If the initial response is good and the LOS resolves, *and* decreasingly small doses of the inotropic agent are needed, there is little likelihood of myocardial damage occurring. However, if the cardiac output can only be maintained by a continuing high or increasing dose, or in the presence of a tachycardia, myocardial damage will inevitably occur and inotropic agents should be avoided.

Afterload reduction

With a failing heart, LOS and a worrying response to inotropic agents there is a further physiological variable to be manipulated with good effect, namely the 'afterload'. This term applies to the stress which is developed in the left ventricular wall during systole. This stress is the major determinant of oxygen consumption, and yet as it increases in quantity it causes an impairment of contraction in the muscle. The stress in the left ventricular wall develops in the period between the mitral valve closing and the aortic valve opening – the period of 'isometric' contraction – and when the aortic valve opens and cardiac emptying begins the stress rapidly diminishes. Thus the quantity of stress will be affected by the pressure at which the aortic valve opens. Consequently, the lower the aortic pressure, the lower the stress in the wall of the left ventricle and the greater the subsequent mechanical contraction of the muscle. This means that if the central aortic pressure is lowered the afterload and oxygen consumption are reduced and at the same time cardic output is improved. This is the theoretical justification for the *vasodilator* treatment of cardiogenic LOS.

In clinical practice, afterload reduction is effective in all its theoretical possibilities provided the arterial pressure is not reduced below a level at which coronary filling is impaired. There are two ways of achieving afterload reduction. The usual way is by vasodilators and, less commonly, by the intra-aortic balloon pump.

Pharmacological reduction of afterload

In low cardiac output, the peripheral resistance rises and tends to maintain the arterial blood pressure. The peripheral resistance is situated at arteriolar level and in order to lower the aortic pressure arteriolar vasodilators are used. Many drugs are suitable for this purpose but ideally should be very short acting and of a predictable action. Nitroprusside and nitroglycerin infusions have these characteristics. Sodium nitroprusside is the more commonly used. During the use of an arteriolar vasodilator, it is important to measure both right and left atrial pressures, aortic pressure and cardiac output by the methods described above.

The drug is infused centrally in a controlled manner and the response of the cardiovascular system monitored. The initial response is for a small fall in central aortic pressure to be followed by an increase in cardiac output. At the same time, because of the vasodilatation some increase in the volume of the circulatory system will occur and lead to lowering of the atrial pressures. The atrial pressure on the left should be restored to 15 mmHg by infusion of either plasma or blood and this usually leads to a further increase in cardiac output. The amount of nitroprusside being infused may be limited by the arterial pressure falling below 70 mmHg systolic or by the development of a tachycardia. These occurrences, however, are infrequent. Pharmacological reduction of the afterload in this manner produces benefits which can easily be demonstrated and yet which seem to defy common sense, i.e. an improvement in cardiac output and action is achieved at a reduced cost to the heart and at the same time peripheral tissue perfusion is increased as a result of the improved cardiac output and vasodilatation.

Intra-aortic ballon pumping (IABP). Reduction in afterload and improved perfusion may be obtained mechanically in those patients who develop an unacceptably low arterial pressure or a tachycardia using pharmacological agents. Intra-aortic balloon pumping (or counter-pulsation) is therefore useful in patients whose cardiac output is extremely low.

Principle of IABP. A balloon is positioned in the descending aorta, having been inserted via the femoral artery (Fig. 5.4). It has a volume of either 30 or 40 ml and is inflated and deflated intermittently using helium. The deflation and inflation are timed to coincide with the cardiac action – inflation of the balloon occurs just as the aortic valve closes at the end of systole and deflation occurs just before the aortic valve opens at the beginning of systolic ejection from the left ventricle.

The effect of inflation is that of a sudden infusion into the ascending aorta of either 30 or 40 ml of blood. The diastolic pressure rises and tissue perfusion, including myocardial perfusion, increases.

When the balloon collapes, the effect is that of withdrawing from the ascending aorta the same amount of blood. This reduces the aortic pressure and permits earlier opening of the aortic

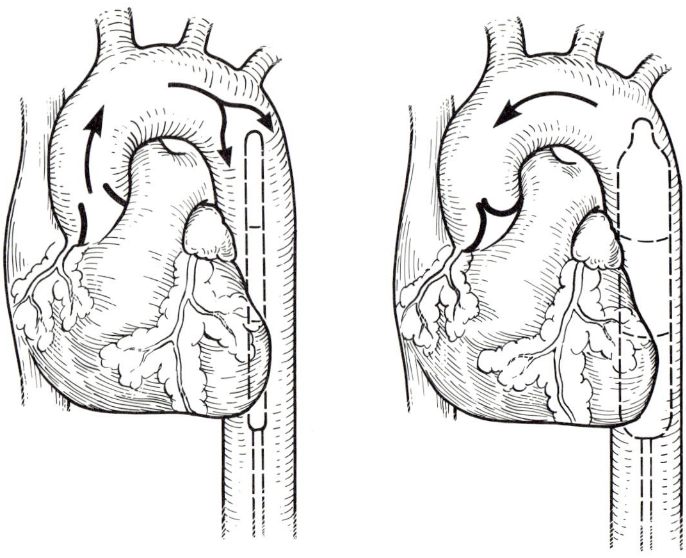

Figure 5.4 Principle of intra-aortic counter-pulsation (IABP).

valve at a lower pressure within the left ventricle. Thus the left ventricular afterload and oxygen consumption are reduced and myocardial contractility improved. In this way the systolic and diastolic blood pressure become reversed with systolic falling below the diastolic.

Clearly, the timing of the pumping is crucial and a large part of the balloon pump console is concerned with this. The pump is activated by the electrical signal of the R wave of the electrocardiograph. Inflation is adjusted so that it begins at the dicrotic notch of the arterial pulse wave and deflation occurs just before the upstroke of the arterial pressure.

Insertion of the balloon. This is an invasive procedure. Under local or general anaesthetic, the common femoral artery is exposed and controlled with atraumatic clamps. The artery is opened longitudinally for about 1 cm and an 8 mm Dacron cuff sewn onto the incision so as to form an artificial side branch to the femoral artery (Fig. 5.5). The balloon is then passed retrogradely so that its tip lies just distal to the origin of the left subclavian artery. The artificial side branch of Dacron is then firmly tied around the tubing of the balloon, the controlling clamps on the artery are released and perfusion of the leg is restarted.

The balloon is then attached to the pump and IABP commenced. The beneficial effects of IABP are usually apparent within a few minutes. The support may be continued for up to three weeks. If left in for more than 24 hours, however, heparinization is necessary to prevent clot forming on the balloon.

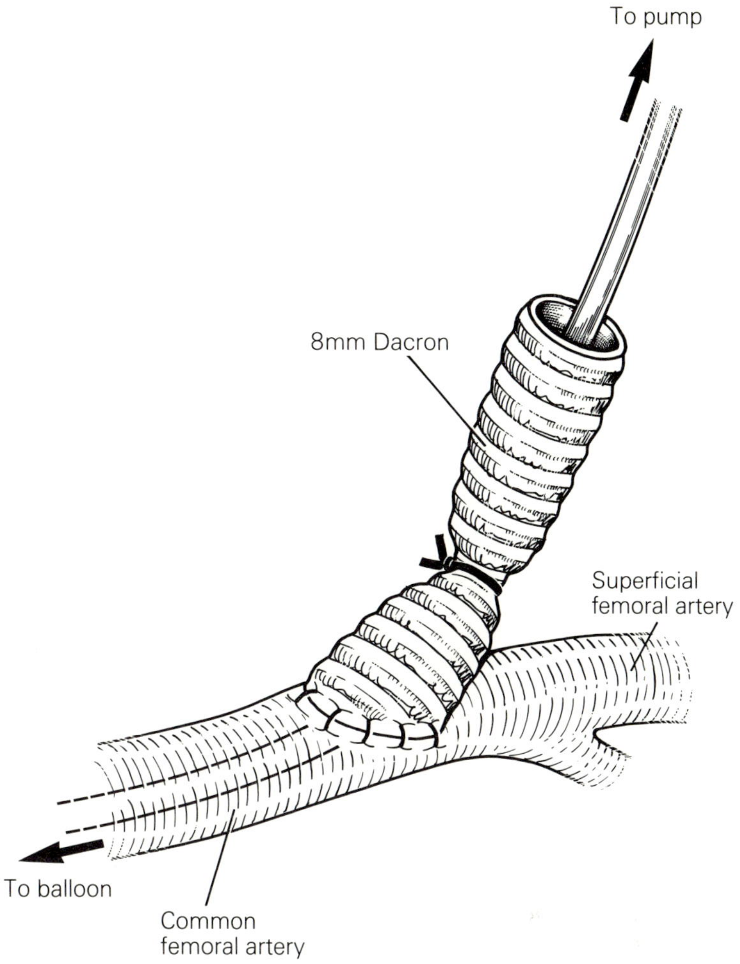

Figure 5.5
One method of insertion of the intra-aortic balloon. The artificial side branch allows the perfusion of the native artery to be unimpeded.

Problems of IABP

1 *Difficulty in inserting the balloon.* This is nearly always due to aortoiliac atheroma. If it is encountered, the other femoral artery should be explored but often the disease is bilateral. Forced passage of the balloon will lead to rupture or dissection of the aorta. If the chest is open, the balloon may be inserted via the ascending aorta but the other manipulations which have been described are not very useful. Peripheral arterial disease may thus prevent the balloon being used.

2 *Damage to the femoral artery* may occur because of disease in it or because the artery is too small to allow passage of the balloon. The ideal solution is to avoid the problem but once it has occurred a vein graft is the best means of restoring perfusion to the leg.

3 *Ischaemic damage to the leg.* This usually happens because of

thrombosis either at the site of insertion or around the stalk of the balloon. The complication is recognized earlier if continuous recording of the temperatures of both feet is made. As the foot cools down with the deficient circulation, it is at first painful and later anaesthetic. Eventually, the muscles of the leg go into spasm and irreversible tissue damage occurs.

Prevention can never be fully effective in the presence of a foreign body lying in an artery. Heparinization will reduce the tendency to thrombosis.

Treatment consists of removing the balloon. If the cardiac output still needs support, some other port of entry must be used. Once ischaemic damage has occurred, early fasciotomy may reduce the tension in the muscle compartments to allow some return of tissue perfusion.

Delay in removing the balloon will lead to loss of the leg. The attending surgeon is therefore faced with a dilemma when confronted by a balloon-dependent patient with an ischaemic leg. Removal of the balloon will threaten the patient's life and leaving it will threaten the leg. There is no clear answer since the individual wishes and circumstances of the patient are unique in every case.

4 *Weaning off the balloon.* As the condition of the patient improves, the need for support will become less. There are controls on the balloon console which permit inflation to be varied from every beat down to one beat in eight. Provided the indirect and direct indices of cardiac output remain stable, the IABP support is reduced through one in two and one in four down to one inflation with every eight cardiac cycles. At this lowest rate, there is no haemodynamic effect on the heart and the intermittent inflation helps to prevent thrombosis around the balloon.

5 *Removal of the balloon.* This is accomplished by reopening the groin and again controlling the artery. The Dacron cuff is trimmed, leaving a 5 mm cuff attached to the artery. The balloon and distal cuff are then removed. Fogarty embolectomy catheters are then passed both proximally and distally to remove thrombi. The cuff is then sewn to prevent blood loss and the flow to the leg restarted. The groin incision is closed.

Occasionally, infection will occur around the Dacron cuff remnant. Antibiotics will not resolve this condition and the cuff should be removed and replaced with a vein patch.

Summary

Low output syndrome after cardiac surgery is managed along conventional lines but is usually multifactorial in origin. Hypovolaemia is sought for and treated first. After that, mechanical causes of cardiac embarrassment are removed. The treatment of myocardial failure is difficult because further damage may be inflicted by inotropic drugs.

Persisting controversies

- Place of exploratory operation in suspected tamponade.
- Indications for vasodilator treatment.
- Indications for IABP.

Bleeding and Cardiac Surgery

Most cardiac operations can be performed with a very low blood loss and many patients do not require blood transfusion during their hospital stay. Obviously all cardiac operations carry the risk of severe bleeding and it is usual for bleeding to be due to a variety of causes, some of which are peculiar to cardiac surgery.

Causes of haemorrhage

Surgical The performance of the operation causes the haemorrhage because, without trauma, no bleeding would occur. The precision with which tissues are divided and cared for will influence the amount of bleeding.

Cardiopulmonary bypass This procedure deranges the clotting mechanisms in a variety of ways, some of which are poorly understood. In the few operations which can be performed either with or without bypass, such as resection of the descending aorta, the amount of bleeding can be shown to be much greater if bypass is used. The clotting mechanism is damaged in a number of ways during bypass:

1 Damage to the labile proteins of the clotting cascade. This occurs as a reaction in the trauma of pumping the blood within the roller pump or at the gas–fluid junction occurring when gases are mixed with the blood. This process is inevitable in a bubble oxygenator and during suction of heparinized shed blood back to the oxygenator.
2 Damage to the platelets during bypass. The numbers and function of platelets become diminished as the bypass lengthens and it is usual for the number of platelets to be as low as 40% of normal afterwards. In certain long bypasses, the level may fall very low. In addition, the function of platelets becomes reduced.
3 'Minor' antigen–antibody reactions occurring in donor–recipient blood, particularly in those cases where fresh donor blood is used in the pump prime. Most adult cases are now operated on with a non-blood prime and this has led to a reduction of bleeding from this cause.
4 Occasionally excessive fibrinolytic activity occurs after cardiopulmonary bypass.

Other causes Pre-existing conditions may cause bleeding after cardiac surgery. Cyanosis causes an impairment of clotting interference at several levels and infection has a similar effect. Many patients are treated with anticoagulants as part of their medical regimen and the effects of these may persist long enough to cause problems at the time of operation. Certain antiplatelet drugs such as dipyridamole and aspirin may have been given. There may be a disturbance of clotting due to a chronic disorder such as Willebrand–Jürgens' syndrome or an acute disorder may follow a viral infection.

Prevention of haemorrhage

Although bleeding after surgery can be helped by blood transfusion, the patient is much better if no bleeding occurs at all and the necessity for transfusion is avoided.

Preoperative prevention

Before the operation a full, haematological screening should take place. The patient's blood group should be determined, along with the haemoglobin level, white cell count and the platelet count. In addition, a full clotting screen is performed and a bleeding time estimated. Any deficiencies in the clotting or bleeding times should lead to the operation being postponed until a specific remedy is available. The commonest problem is a deficiency of platelets, the cause for this being usually unclear although viral infections have been thought to be a major cause.

Oral anticoagulants should be stopped before surgery if possible and laboratory estimations of the prothrombin time made. If urgent surgery has to be performed on a patient taking anticoagulants up to the time of surgery, 20 mg of vitamin K by intramuscular injection are given four hours before operation and fresh frozen plasma should be made available afterwards.

Some patients, especially those with cyanosis, infection or having a second operation, are greatly at risk from bleeding. In such patients, the blood bank should be informed several days before the operation and fresh blood should be available for transfusion (see below).

Perioperative prevention

The skill and care of the surgeon will help to prevent much of the bleeding. As the chest wall is being opened, usually by a median sternotomy, careful control of all bleeding points is performed by diathermy. The sternum is opened by an electric saw and specific bleeding points in the periosteum controlled by diathermy. Bleeding from the medulla of the sternum is generally ignored but specific troublesome points are controlled with bone wax. However, too much wax will cause impaired bony healing.

The sternotomy incision is opened gradually as the deeper tissues are divided in order to avoid shearing of the various tissue planes causing bleeding. Most bleeding in a median sternotomy incision is caused by wandering away from the midline of the chest wall.

The pericardium is opened and any thymic remnants should be ligated and then divided. If adhesions are present in the pericardium, they should be precisely divided with scissors. Increased bleeding is *not* caused by division of adhesions themselves but by trauma to the tissues which the adhesions join. In other words, precise division which does not damage the underlying or overlying tissues will not cause excessive bleeding. The temptation to 'sweep away' adhesions with a swab or finger should be avoided for this reason. If adhesions are present, sufficient of the dissection should be performed to allow cannulation and cardiopulmonary bypass to be started. Once the heart is empty and ventilation stopped, the dissection becomes much easier. The ideal conditions for dissection are found when the heart is paralysed and collapsed after cardioplegia has been instituted. Consequently, if cardioplegia is to be used it should be given as soon as bypass can be established and the ascending aorta cross-clamped.

The surgical technique of closing cardiac incisions is important for the prevention of haemorrhage. Cardiac incisions are made into the muscle of the ventricles or into the thinner walled atria or great vessels. In muscle incisions, closure is achieved by accurate approximation of the muscle using interrupted unabsorbable sutures which are fairly thick (say 2/0). The tension needed to approximate the edges is diminished if the heart is decompressed. Too high a tension will cause the suture to cut through the tissue. If this should happen, the suture must be buttressed with a pledget of Teflon felt or similar material and placed as a horizontal mattress suture.

Incisions in the atria or great vessels are repaired by means of an everting continuous suture using a thin (3/0) monofilament material on an atraumatic round-bodied needle. The first layer of everting suture is then reinforced with a continuous over-and-over suture placed *externally* to the first layer.

The suture line is satisfactory if no bleeding occurs through it at normal pressures and with full heparinization. Extra sutures may be needed, especially in aortic suture lines, and under these circumstances the pressure within the aorta should be lowered to prevent the suture cutting through the tissue. Such a reduction in pressure may be achieved by the use of drugs or by temporarily cross-clamping the inferior vena cava if the patient is supporting his own circulation. If on bypass, the pump flow should be reduced to a very low level for the few seconds it takes to insert and tie the stitch.

At the end of the operation, the chest should not be closed until there is evidence of minimal bleeding. Every suture line and cardiac incision should be checked and every point of the extracardiac tissues examined and re-examined. There should be evidence of firm clot due to protamine reversal of heparin.

The sternum is usually closed with wire sutures passing through the halves of the bone and danger to the internal mammary artery exists. Each wire should be inspected; if there is any doubt of internal mammary artery bleeding, control should be achieved with an undermining unabsorbable stitch. Diathermy alone will not control an internal mammary artery for long.

Most surgical teams reverse heparin by giving three times the calculated reversal dose of protamine. This is usually satisfactory but accurate and repeated heparin–protamine neutralization tests will lead to more precise control of heparin activity. Semiautomatic machines which may be used in the operating theatre are available but are expensive to use.

Haemostasis at the end of a long operation is tedious and often neglected by a tired surgeon but attention at this time, often by a second surgeon who is fresh, will pay handsomely. A few minutes extra in ensuring adequate haemostasis may save several hours of surgical time in the night following operation.

Summary Care taken during the operation will help to reduce bleeding. Accurate closure of cardiac incisions and division of adhesions is necessary. Care and time must be spent after the cardiac part of the operation to ensure that no surgical bleeding will persist. Bleeding after an operation would not occur unless an operation had been performed, and surgical control of bleeding is the first requirement to avoid haemorrhage after the operation.

Persisting controversy

- Operating theatre control of the reversal of heparin by protamine is crude and more accurate reversal will help to reduce haemorrhage.

Treatment of haemorrhage during and after cardiac surgery

During the operation the chest is not closed unless the amount of bleeding is small and there is obvious clot formation. Thus the only danger of haemorrhage in the operating theatre is that of exsanguination and this is avoided by blood transfusion.

If the surgeon is confident that there is no hole which is bleeding, the bleeding must be due to a deficiency of haemostasis. At the outset, it needs to be said that the judgement of the surgeon may be wrong due to a variety of causes such as an inaccessible bleeding point or surgical fatigue. Therefore, the surgeon must never assume that there is no surgical lesion causing the bleeding until the situation is controlled. Repeated inspections, particularly of the back of the heart, are essential.

In the meantime, samples are sent to the coagulation laboratory for detailed investigation of clotting function. If a specific factor of the clotting mechanism is deranged, then the specific treatment should be given. This is often but not always effective. Specific component therapy is very popular on many units, possibly more with haematologists than with surgeons. Many haematologists believe that the answer to clotting disorders is to identify the disorder precisely and give the precise component to remedy that disorder. Many surgeons are sceptical of such an approach. They remember patients who did not form clot in spite of no demonstrable laboratory evidence of abnormality and they have seen various theories of normal clotting discarded as new facts have emerged. These surgeons would prefer to give patients fresh blood as treatment. The rationale for this that platelet function in fresh blood is good and there are many times when fresh blood works and component therapy does not. There is no clear answer to this controversy and each unit must evolve its own policy which depends on many factors, both medical and logistical.

After the operation, bleeding is doubly dangerous. The danger of exsanguination persists and there is the added problem of cardiac tamponade. It is important after operation to appreciate that while various clotting abnormalities may be present, the bleeding would not be happening if the patient had not undergone an operation. Any bleeding after surgery is therefore assumed to be surgical in the first instance. That assumption leads inevitably to the attitude that excessive bleeding after surgery will probably only be controlled by further surgery. A second operation will be indicated immediately on most units if the bleeding exceeds more than 500 ml in any one hour in an adult patient. Smaller volumes are acceptable in children according to their size. An expectant attitude towards heavy bleeding is to be deplored. 'All bleeding stops eventually' is a surgical dictum which is very useful.

If the bleeding is heavy, but does not exceed the volumes stated above, a wait of an hour or two may be justifiable unless tamponade occurs. A clotting screen may reveal a treatable abnormality. The arterial blood pressure may be reduced from an excessively high level by drugs such as nitroprusside. Use of positive end-expiratory pressure (PEEP) via the ventilator may reduce mediastinal bleeding. If these manoeuvres are not effective within an hour or two, however, the patient should undergo a second operation to stop the bleeding and to prevent tamponade.

Re-exploration for bleeding is ideally performed within a few hours of the first operation. The benefits are that bleeding is usually controlled before excessive transfusion is needed and the danger of tamponade is removed. Often, at the second operation, a surprising degree of cardiac compression may be found. Delay in reoperating carries no advantages and many dangers, and is usually inconveniently timed in the small hours of the morning on a very sick patient.

Summary

Bleeding after cardiac surgery is usually due to surgical causes. Only when these have been excluded should abnormalities of clotting be blamed. Re-exploration should be performed immediately if the haemorrhage exceeds 500 ml in one hour or 300 ml an hour for three or more consecutive hours. Re-exploration should be undertaken more readily in cases which are bleeding less severely if simple measures fail.

Persisting controversies

- Use and indications for fresh blood.
- Liberal indications for re-exploration in bleeding after cardiac surgery.

Conclusion

Bleeding after cardiac surgery may be due to several causes including impaired clotting and the nature of the cardiac disorder. However, surgical trauma is the precipitating event and the attention of the surgeon should be directed towards minimizing and then treating this particular cause before anything else (see flow diagram opposite). Re-exploration for bleeding should be performed early when indications are right, and procrastination should be avoided.

Brain Damage

The lack of any capacity for anaerobic respiration in nerve cells causes them to be extremely vulnerable to the effects of inadequate oxygen supply. During cardiac surgery and afterwards, there are many factors which may cause brain damage by hypoxia. Brain damage is the most common serious complication of open-heart surgery (Table 5.1).

Detection of brain damage

The amount of brain damage may vary enormously. One patient may have total brain death and another merely some confusion, temporary loss of memory or perhaps a subtle alteration of concentration only noticeable to the patient himself. Many studies have been performed to assess the numbers of patients having this complication after cardiac surgery. It is clear that the number depends on the criteria for brain damage which are

Table 5.1
Causes of brain damage during cardiac surgery.

1 *Small cerebral vessel occlusion by emboli*
  (a) Air
  (b) Debris from the heart, operative site, or heart–lung machine
  (c) Aggregated blood cells

2 *Inadequate total flow*
  (a) Cardiac arrest
  (b) Inadequate output from the heart–lung machine during bypass
  (c) Carotid artery disease

3 *Cerebral haemorrhage*

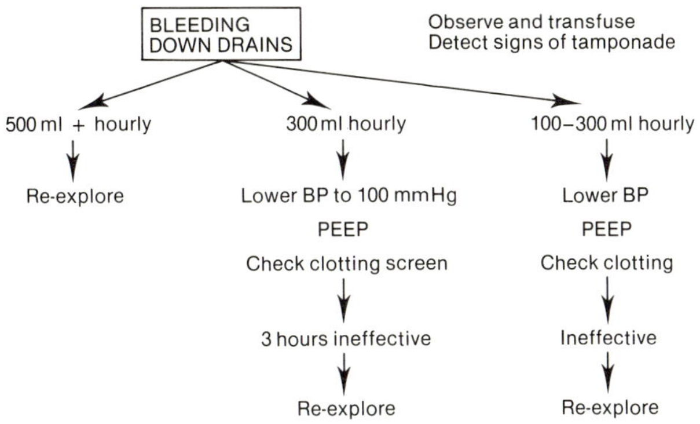

Management of the bleeding patient after cardiac surgery

applied. If only gross objective neurological damage is accepted, then about 0.5–1% of patients having open-heart surgery will be diagnosed as having brain damage. However, if the criteria are more subtle and expanded to include less objective signs, such as confusion or impairment of certain intellectual functions, then perhaps 8–10% of patients are at risk. Not even these criteria, however, will include those patients with altered personality or concentration not detectable by psychological tests. Those surgeons who make careful neurological assessments before and after surgery will invariably report a higher incidence of brain damage. Those surgeons who record an electroencephalogram during and after operation will have the highest incidence of all.

General methods of prevention of brain damage
The patient about to have cardiac surgery should always have a full neurological examination. This should include the palpation and auscultation of the carotid arteries in the neck to detect lesions which might cause problems during operation. Any abnormality here should lead to Doppler examination of the carotid arteries. Angiography may follow if indicated.

Some patients have had cerebrovascular accidents before surgery. Depending on the urgency of cardiac surgery, it is desirable to avoid operation for about a month after such incidents because their manifestations become more severe, possibly due to oedema or haemorrhage. Even several months afterwards, when full or partial recovery has taken place, neurological signs may worsen (for a while) immediately after surgery. Obviously, cardiac arrest at any time should be avoided to prevent brain damage.

Embolic brain damage
This most often occurs after open-heart surgery but may complicate such operations as closed mitral valvotomy. Any embolus capable of blocking the immediate precapillary arterioles will

cause brain damage. Therefore the size of embolus necessary to be damaging may be anything from about 15 μm upwards. The nature and amount of neurological damage will depend on the types and numbers of brain arteries or arterioles which become occluded. Whether or not the embolus is capable of being absorbed is not usually important because neurological damage occurs so quickly.

Causes of embolic brain damage

1 *Air bubbles* (discussed in detail on page 103).
2 *Emboli due to debris.* The operative site, including the towels, the heart and the whole of the heart–lung machine, are areas from which debris may enter the arterial circulation. Calcium particles, thrombus from the left atrium, pericardial fat globules and even fragments of suture material have been described as emboli.
3 *Emboli due to aggregated blood cells.* During cardiopulmonary bypass, a large number of physiological disturbances affect the patient's blood: the tubing and oxygenator are foreign surfaces; the oxygenator is probably a 'bubble' type (see Fig. 6.4) and causes an air–fluid interface; and the pumping system is traumatic and causes non-pulsatile flow. In addition, donor blood may be added during bypass and although it may be compatible on ABO and Rhesus criteria, other more subtle incompatibilities may be present. As a result of all these factors, and others which are less well understood, a tendency is created for red cells and platelets to form clusters which vary in size from 15 to 100 μm. These 'microemboli' are always present during cardiopulmonary bypass and cause dysfunction of all tissues eventually. As usual, the brain is the first organ to suffer.

Prevention of embolic brain damage

1 *Air.* Removal of air from the heart at the end of bypass is the responsibility of the operating surgeon and, as already stated, there are many techniques. These are discussed fully on page 103.
2 *Particulate microemboli,* whether composed of debris or aggregated blood cells, are not so directly under the surgeon's control. All shed heparinized blood which is sucked back to the heart–lung circuit should be filtered through a pore size of 15 μm. Many surgeons place such filters in the arterial line leading back to the patient but others believe that microemboli may result from placing filters in the arterial line. Larger pore filters of up to 150 μm are incorporated at other places in the extracorporeal circuit.

Summary

Embolic brain damage is caused by air or particulate emboli. Air embolus is a preventable hazard and is under the surgeon's control. Particulate emboli are inevitable and large screen and microfiltration should be inserted in the extracorporeal circulation.

Persisting controversies

- The ideal way to remove 'surgical' air.
- The placement of microfilters in the extracorporeal circulation.

Brain damage due to inadequate total flow

Cardiac arrest, by definition, leads to an inadequate brain blood flow. Carotid artery lesions may escape detection before surgery but may reduce blood flow significantly at the lower pressures to be found during cardiopulmonary bypass. These causes are self evident. Less clear, however, is the pressure at which the brain must be perfused during bypass. The issue is complicated because of the non-pulsatile flow and the reduction of temperature of the perfusate and the body.

During cardiopulmonary bypass, many surgeons prefer to restrict the output from the machine is order to achieve better operating conditions. The carbon dioxide tension in the perfusing fluid will also determine the state of dilatation of the cerebral blood vessels. Consequently, it is a far from simple matter to know how much pressure and flow the brain needs to remain undamaged.

Prevention of damage due to inadequate flow

Clearly, cardiac arrest should be avoided if at all possible and treated vigorously when it occurs. Similarly, carotid artery lesions should be sought for and if significant may need surgery before or during the heart operation.

The balance of evidence suggests that a perfusion pressure of around 50 mmHg is sufficient to preserve the brain tissue, if the perfusion is conducted at the calculated flow for that patient and assuming a moderate degree of hypothermia (32–34 °C). Simple electroencephalograms ('cerebral function monitors') are used during the bypass in some centres with good effect. Others prefer not to use cerebral function monitors because of difficulties in interpretation and electrical interference in the operating threatre.

Summary

Brain damage due to inadequate flow may be prevented by treating significant carotid artery lesions and perfusing at a pressure of at least 50 mmHg during cardiopulmonary bypass.

Persisting controversy

- Use of cerebral function monitors during cardiopulmonary bypass.

Treatment of established brain damage after cardiac surgery

Once cerebral damage occurs, the effects will be due to both reversible and irreversible lesions. The object of treatment is to prevent further cells becoming damaged by oedema and intracranial swelling.

The first sign of cerebral damage after cardiac surgery is failure to regain consciousness and to obey simple commands.

Once it is clear that this is not due to residual anaesthetic, treatment is begun with an anti-inflammatory steroid. Dexamethasone, 8 mg immediately i.v. and 4 mg eight-hourly thereafter for three days, is usually used in some units.

Thereafter, all that one can do is wait for recovery to occur. There are no quick ways to hasten recovery from a cerebral insult. In the meantime, full support for the patient must be given. Air embolic damage often recovers surprisingly quickly but may often be disappointingly incomplete.

Flexion contractures in the limbs should be prevented by passive limb movements. Care of the unconscious or confused, cerebrally damaged patient is often made easy by a tracheostomy. Epilepsy occurring during the recovery period of a cerebral injury should be treated with the appropriate anticonvulsants. Merely to paralyse and sedate the patient is insufficient.

Summary The prevention of cerebral damage during cardiac surgery is much more important than the treatment of the established lesion. No specific measures are available apart from the use of dexamethasone.

Conclusion

Cerebral damage after cardiac surgery is the major cause of mortality and morbidity. Since no specific treatment is available, prevention must be emphasized. Removal of 'surgical' air should be given its proper importance. All bypass circuits should contain not only large screen filters but also microfilters in order to prevent particulate brain embolism.

Further Reading

Branthwaite, M.A. (1975) Prevention of neurological damage during open heart surgery. *Thorax, 30*, 258–261.

Cohn, J.N. & Franciosa, J.A. (1977) Vasodilator therapy of heart failure. *N. Engl. J. Med., 297*, 27–31, 254–258.

Conti, V.R., Bertranou, E.G., Blackstone, E.H., Kirklin, J.W. & Digerness, S.B. (1978) Cold cardioplegia versus hypothermia for myocardial protection. *J. Thorac. Cardiovasc. Surg., 76*, 577–589.

Follette, D.M., Fey, K., Mulder, D.M., Maloney, J.V. & Buckberg, G.D. (1977) Prolonged safe aortic cross clamping by combining membrane stabilization multidose cardioplegia and physiologic reperfusion. *J. Thorac. Cardiovasc. Surg., 74*, 682.

Gay, W.A., Jr & Ebert, P.A. (1973) Functional, metabolic and morphologic effects of K induced cardioplegia. *Surgery, 74*, 284.

Hoffman, J.I.E. & Buckberg, G.D. (1975) Contemporary themes. Pathophysiology of sub-endocardial ischaemia. *Br. Med. J., i*, 76–79.

Maloney, J.V., Cooper, N., Mulder, D.G. & Buckberg, G.D. (1975) Depressed cardiac perfusion after mitral valve replacement – a problem of myocardial preservation during operation. *Circulation* (Supplement 1), *51 & 52*, 1–3.

Marengo-Rowe, A.J., Lambert, C.J., Mitchel, B.F. et al. (1979) The evaluation of haemorrhage in cardiac patients who have undergone extracorporeal circulation. *Transfusion*, *19*, 62.

McEnany, M.T., Kay, H.R., Buckley, M.J., Daggett, W.M., Erdmann, A.J., Mundth, E.D., Rao, R.S., Detoeut, J. & Austen, W.G. (1978) Clinical experience with IABP support in 728 patients. *Circulation*, *58* (Supplement 1 – Cardiovascular Surgery, 1977).

6 Complications of Cardiopulmonary Bypass

Almost all open-heart operations are carried out using the heart–lung machine which bypasses and substitutes for the functions of the heart and lungs. Regardless of the exact nature of the operation, there are risks and complications of the cardiopulmonary bypass procedure. An understanding of the principles of cardiopulmonary bypass is necessary in order to appreciate the potential hazards. While exact details of technique are unimportant in this context, inevitably some technical hazards will be described.

After the patient has been anaesthetized, the chest is opened. This is usually performed by a vertical split in the midline anteriorly – the median sternotomy. The heart is exposed by dividing the pericardium vertically. In order to remove the venous blood from the circulation, cannulation of the right atrium or both venae cavae is performed. The venous blood is drained by siphonage into the heart–lung machine. In this device, the blood is oxygenated, pumped up to arterial pressure and delivered back to the patient's arterial system whence it may perfuse the systemic circulation. While the bypass is working, the heart no longer delivers blood to the pulmonary or systemic circulations and may be opened, drained of its contents and corrective surgery performed.

At the outset, the artificial nature of the oxygenation and pumping systems must be appreciated. Both systems are less efficient than the heart and lungs, and additionally create damage. There is a limited time during which cardiopulmonary bypass may be tolerated. The normal cardiac operation can usually be done in less than two hours of bypass, but bypass lasting longer than four hours is associated with a rapidly increasing incidence of mortality and morbidity. Modern cardiopulmonary bypass, however, is more commonly complicated by avoidable surgical hazards rather than problems due to the physiological inadequacy of equipment. Failure to provide an adequate flow of arterial blood to the body will first cause brain damage because of its sensitivity to hypoxia.

Avoidable Surgical Hazards (Table 6.1)

Arterial air embolism

Air in the arterial circulation will cause permanent damage to the brain and temporary damage to other organs including the heart. Cerebral damage from arterial air embolism is the most common cause of morbidity and mortality in modern cardiac surgery. Estimates of its incidence vary from 2 to 20%; around 5% of patients having cardiopulmonary bypass will have some evidence of permanent neurological damage; far fewer will be in any way troubled by such damage.

The source of the air lies in the opened drained heart. As the cardiac repair is accomplished and the heart begins again to support a circulation, steps must be taken by the surgeon in order to replace all the air with blood. The nature of the anatomy inside the heart provides many places in which air may become trapped only to embolize later, common places being the left atrial appendage and the spaces between muscle bundles inside the left ventricle. The difficulty of removing air from such places, and the fact that such a small volume of air (probably 1–2 ml) in the cerebral circulation may cause severe damage, leads surgeons to become very careful about 'degassing' the heart during bypass.

Every surgeon has his preferred technique but the total evacuation of air is an impossibility. Techniques which allow the heart to beat, thus expelling air along with blood, are more effective than techniques performed with the flaccid heart. All techniques involve the removal of air and blood from the left atrium, left ventricle and aorta. Suction applied to each of these chambers will help the process. Massaging the pulmonary veins will dislodge air trapped there (Fig. 6.1). However, no matter what technique is applied, several minutes are probably necessary for its full effectiveness, and even then most surgeons assume that some air will escape into the systemic circulation. In order to avoid cerebral vessel occlusion, a steep head-down position of the patient will aid the passage of air into less vulnerable tissues.

Even when the heart has supported a circulation for several minutes, some entrapped air may be dislodged from its cavities and pass into the ascending aorta and thus to the systemic

Table 6.1 Hazards of cardiopulmonary bypass.

Avoidable surgical hazards
1 Arterial air embolism
2 Bleeding
3 Cannulation of the great vessels

Unavoidable hazards of the procedure
1 Problems of priming fluids
2 Problems of the oxygenator
3 Problems of the pump

Figure 6.1
One method of evacuating air from the left ventricle. The system works most effectively with a beating heart.

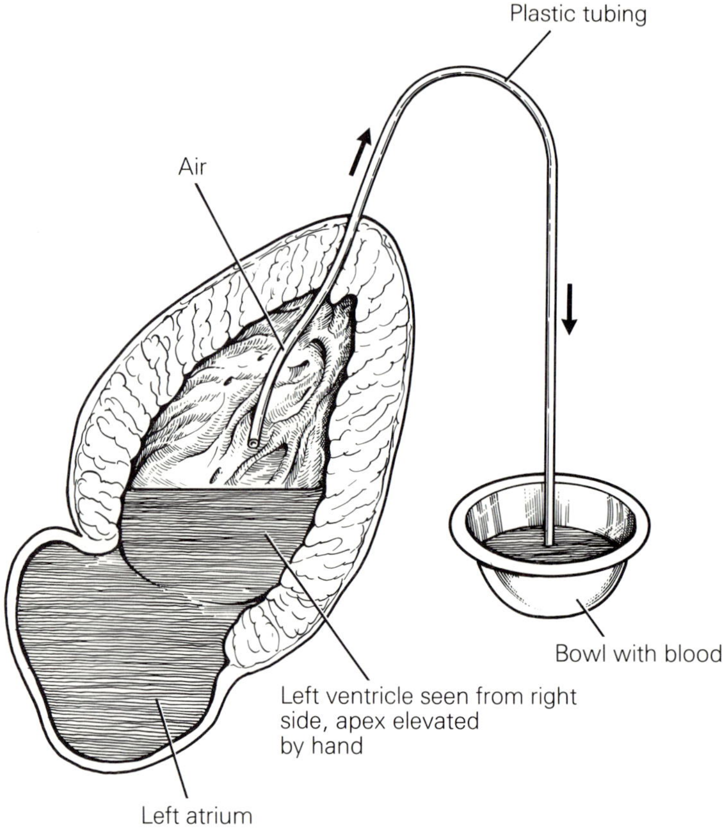

circulation. A cannula placed in the highest part of the aorta and gently sucking blood from it to the heart–lung machine will help to reduce this hazard. A partial occlusion clamp placed on the aorta just dowstream of this site will form a little 'cupola' and will increase the efficiency of this technique to remove residual air (Fig. 6.2). Any air coming from the left ventricle will rise into the cupola and escape through the venting needle.

Air in the coronary circulation is a hazard which causes severe myocardial depression and thus a longer period of cardiac support. Long-term damage from air has been described. Usually the emboli are absorbed within a few minutes and the coronary circulation returns to normal.

Cerebral air embolism always causes neurological damage (see also page 96). Chance will determine if the damage is important or not. Such damage is irreversible and therefore no treatment of the neuronal lesion is possible. Secondary damage by oedema may be minimized by the use of steroid drugs. Obsessive and prolonged attention directed towards the prevention of cerebral air embolism is necessary in each case. Such an attitude can be encouraged in trainee surgeons by placing a Doppler recorder on the carotids of the patient having open-heart surgery. Such a device emits a noise when an air bubble passes up the carotid artery and gives an audible demonstration of the difficulties in preventing this, the most serious complication.

Bleeding

This has already been discussed (page 91).

Cannulation of the great vessels

Cannulation of the heart and great vessels is an integral part of cardiopulmonary bypass. The insertion of wide-bore plastic tubes is a surgical procedure, the risks of which can be diminished by appropriate techniques.

The mainstay of such techniques is the pursestring suture (Fig. 6.3). A circle of tissue (right atrium, vena cava or aorta) about 1.5 cm in diameter is enclosed by stitch of 2/0 polypropylene suture taking several bites, each penetrating the outer one-half to one-third of the wall. The long ends of the stitch are then brought through a rubber snare and clamped so as to enable the stitch to be controllably tightened or loosened. An incision is made between the stitches and the cannula introduced. When the cannula is removed the stitch is tightened and tied. Serious bleeding is rarely encountered in venous cannulation but arterial cannulation is asociated with two hazards.

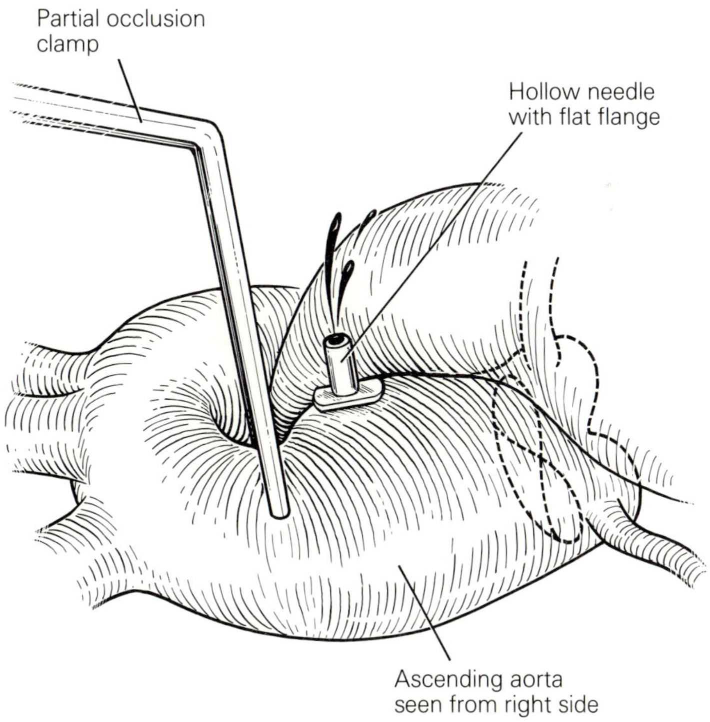

Figure 6.2 One method of removing residual air from the ascendng aorta when the heart is supporting a circulation

Figure 6.3
One method of cannulating the ascending aorta: (a) preparation, (b) snare tightened around cannula (snare and cannula are tied together to prevent displacement of cannula).

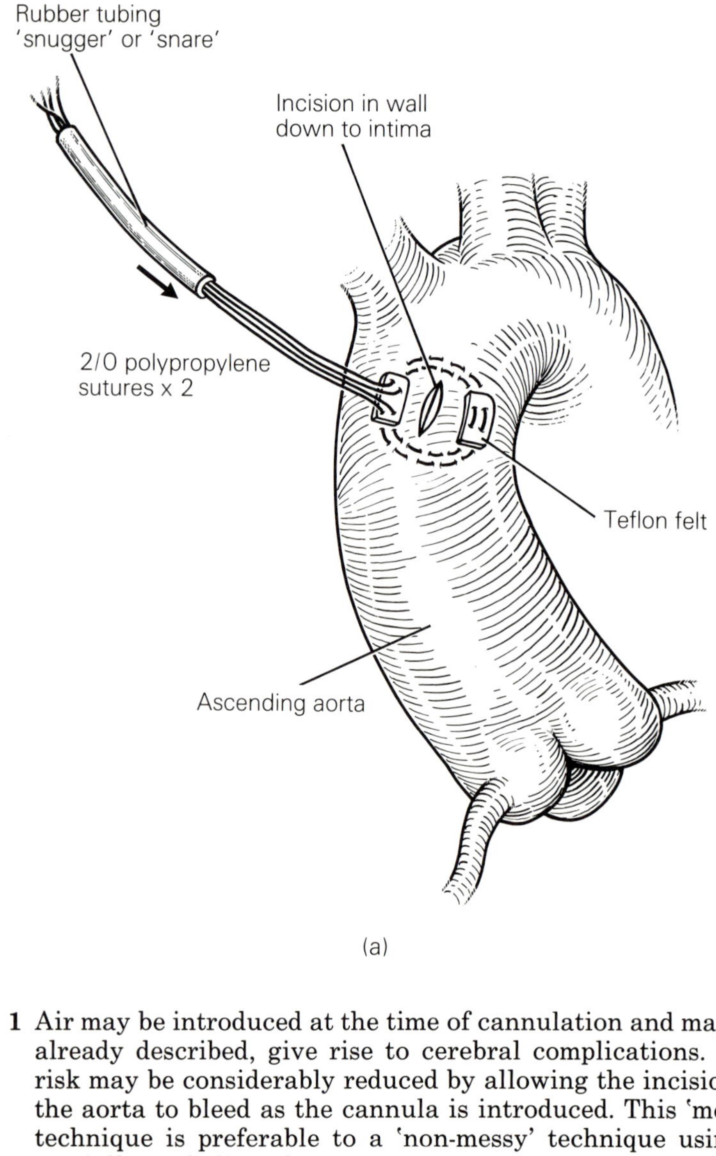

(a)

1 Air may be introduced at the time of cannulation and may, as already described, give rise to cerebral complications. This risk may be considerably reduced by allowing the incision in the aorta to bleed as the cannula is introduced. This 'messy' technique is preferable to a 'non-messy' technique using a partially occluding clamp.

2 Because of the arterial pressure, bleeding may occur when the cannula is removed. This may be due to an extension of the incision, a tear of the suture holes or merely high pressure. Arterial decannulation is best performed with a low arterial pressure. This may be achieved by the administration of drugs by the anaesthetist or by a temporary clamping of the inferior vena cava within the pericardium.

Most bleeding from the cardiac cannulation sites or incisions can be controlled by one or two extra sutures. Should the tissue

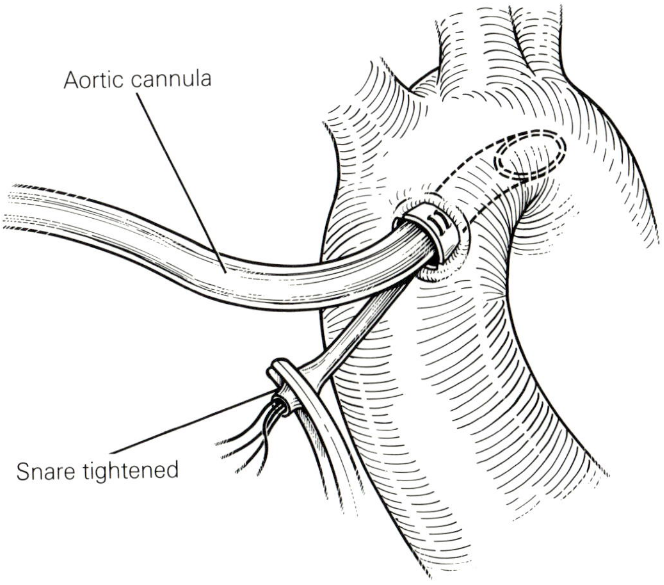

(b)

be friable or the pressure high, however, tearing may occur. This may be prevented or treated by using a buttressed suture technique. Tearing is less likely if a non-absorbable monofilament suture is used.

Unavoidable Hazards of the Procedure

Problems of priming fluids

Pumping mechanisms need to be filled with the fluid they are to move and this process is called 'priming'. The heart–lung machine is no exception and before the patient's blood can be circulated through it, the circuit has to be primed. In the early days of cardiopulmonary bypass fresh blood primes were used, but in spite of all supposition proved to be damaging. Evidence of small vessel damage appeared in many organs after the procedure and this was probably due to complex antigen–antibody reactions. Slowly, blood was replaced by non-blood solutions as the priming fluid and most surgeons now use an entirely crystalloid fluid prime such as Hartmann's solution.

Such a fluid load is between 2 and 3 l and clearly must mix with the patient's own blood as the procedure begins. The consequent dilution of blood leads to very few problems provided the packed cell volume (PCV) is kept above 20%. Below this level, impairment of tissue oxygenation occurs and is reflected in organ dysfunction after the operation.

After bypass, the body elminates most of the prime and restores the packed red cell volume to normal within a few hours. This is achieved by urinary losses mostly, but there is an increase in the total extracellular fluid volume of about 20% which lasts for some days. Many patients are helped by a diuretic to eliminate this extra load.

Once blood is added to the pump prime in order to maintain an adequate PCV, there will be greater difficulty in obtaining haemostasis and usually postoperative blood losses will be higher. Most of this increase can be eliminated by obsessive surgical technique.

If blood is used as a priming fluid, ideally it should be fresh but not so fresh that it contains all the cellular elements of blood. After two to three days, all the white cells and platelets will have disappeared and the blood is ideal for use. However, most surgeons who operate on small children will insist on very fresh blood for priming the cardiopulmonary bypass circuit as the results seem to be better than with other primes.

After the cardiopulmonary bypass, the contents of the heart–lung machine are collected in sterile bags and given back to the patient according to the needs of the circulation. Excess fluid is eliminated by the kidneys and the patient receives back his own red cells.

The use of non-blood primes has been very important in the development of open-heart surgery. Not only have there been important advantages for the patient but the expense and logistical difficulties of providing cardiopulmonary bypass have been greatly reduced, thus making the procedure simpler, quicker and more widely available. With the use of a non-blood prime and careful attention to haemostasis during the operation, it is possible to perform open-heart surgery without the use of donor blood, thus avoiding the known hazards.

Problems of the oxygenator

In the normal individual, blood is oxygenated and carbon dioxide removed by passing through the vast area available for gas transfer in the lungs. Blood and air are always separated by at least the alveolar membrane and never meet. The artificial oxygenator of the cardiopulmonary bypass circuit cannot reach the efficiency and safety of normal lung tissue.

Artificial oxygenators are of two types, depending on the way in which blood is oxygenated. First, the blood may be oxygenated by blowing through it a constant stream of oxygen. This creates a foam in which the blood is oxygenated and loses carbon dioxide. This process is clearly unphysiological in that blood and oxygen mix intimately. Oxygenators employing this method are called 'bubble' oxygenators (Fig. 6.4) and at the time of writing are the most widely used. Alternatively, the oxygenator may consist of a wide area of very thin artificial material which separates blood and oxygen but allows gas diffusion. Such devices are called

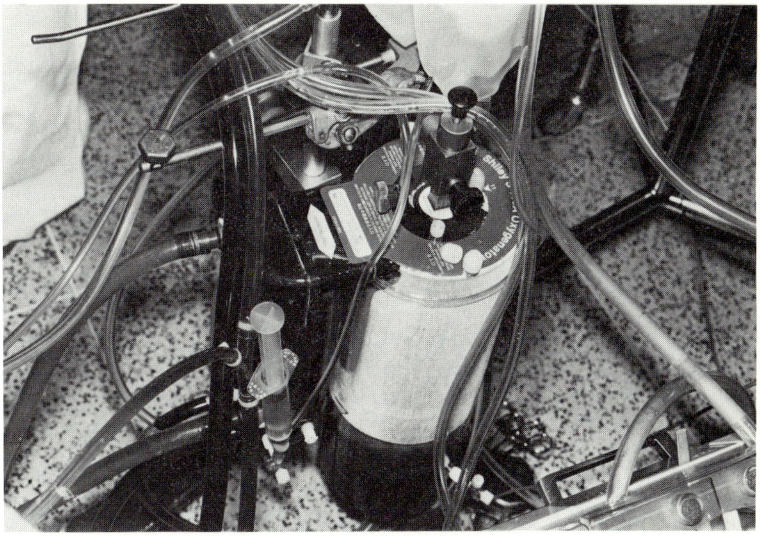

Figure 6.4 Commercially available bubble oxygenator in use.

'membrane' oxygenators (Fig. 6.5) and are clearly more physiological in many respects. They are, however, relatively expensive and relatively inefficient compared with normal lung tissue. The choice between using a membrane or bubble oxygenator is not easy (Table 6.2). Clearly, if a long procedure is expected a membrane oxygenator will offer advantages, particularly if the heart is not going to be opened, with the risk of surgical air embolism being avoided.

However, most cardiac surgical procedures are relatively short and involve opening the heart. The patient is then more at risk from surgical air embolism than from deficiencies in the oxygenator. Accordingly, the decision on whether a bubble or membrane oxygenator should be used is made on consideration of the patient, the nature of the operation and the likely length of the bypass.

Problems of the pump

Blood is a tissue composed of cells in the liquid matrix and is as sensitive to damage as any other tissue. Thus, pumping blood from venous up to arterial pressure and to a near normal cardiac output exposes the blood to a greater or lesser degree of trauma.

During the development of cardiopulmonary bypass, many ingenious devices for pumping blood have been developed, but most have been abandoned because of the damage they caused to the blood. The most widely used pump at present is the roller pump (Fig. 6.6). The electric motor rotates an arm which has rollers on each end. These compress a silicone rubber tube which thus propels blood onward. Provided the rollers are adjusted to provide the least compression necessary to occlude the tube, the level of damage to the blood is acceptable, but poor adjustment of

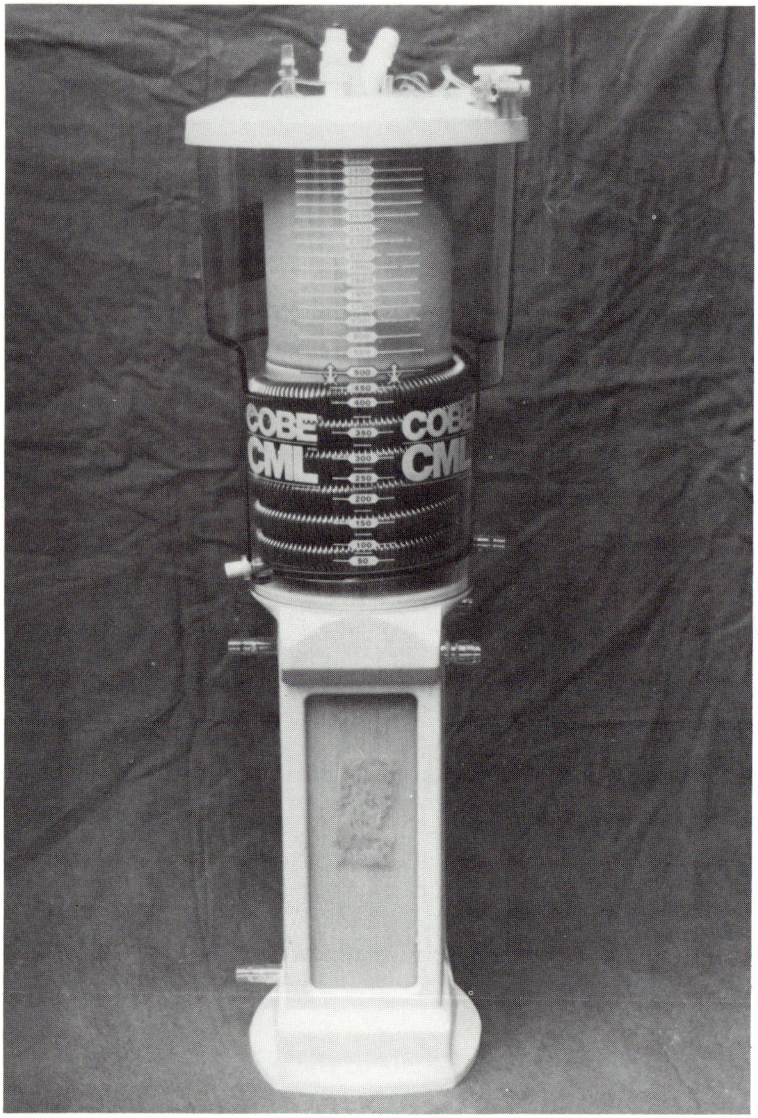

Figure 6.5
Membrane oxygenator.

the rollers, high flows or prolonged periods of pumping will cause detectable blood damage.

The flow of the pump will clearly be determined by the speed of the motor which is varied by the pump operator in order to meet the demands of the patient's body. If the rollers are applied too closely to the silicone rubber tube, it may be split – quite apart from the extra blood trauma. If the rollers do not provide full occlusion of the tubing in the pump, again blood damage will occur, but even more importantly the pump may not be delivering the calculated flow back to the patient causing severe organ damage particularly involving the kidneys.

Table 6.2
Comparison of bubble and membrane oxygenators.

	Bubble oxygenator	*Membrane oxygenator*
Advantages	Simplicity Low cost	Easy to operate No blood–gas interface No disturbance of plasma proteins, platelets or red cells
Disadvantages	Air embolism Effects of blood–gas interface **1** Proteins denatured **2** Fragility of red cells **3** Platelet damage	Expense

Other Avoidable Problems

Suction

During cardiopulmonary bypass the patient is heparinized. Blood shed during the procedure mostly falls into the pericardium. From here, and from inside the cardiac chambers, suction will return blood to the bypass circuit to allow its recirculation. This recycling of the blood which is lost thus reduces the need for blood transfusion.

However, suction damages blood by the forcible aspiration of it and air into the suction tubing. Many of the problems of mixing air and blood will occur, as well as the trauma of suddenly imparting motion to this delicate liquid tissue. In addition, other non-blood substances may be sucked into the circuit at the same time, such as liquid fat and secretions from the pericardium.

Suction damages the blood more than any other part of the cardiopulmonary bypass procedure. While some suction is necessary to allow the operation to be performed, it must be kept as low as possible and any blood which is contaminated by other secretions should be discarded. Damage to the blood by suction will cause haemolysis and haemoglobin in the urine. Platelet function will be excessively diminished and further derange the clotting function of blood.

If excessive quantities of blood are found in the heart and excessive suction is needed, it is probably better to reduce the pump flow and arterial pressure for a while rather than rely on excessive suction.

Microemboli

All the unphysiological events of the cardiopulmonary bypass circuit work together in producing some aggregation of the formed cellular elements of blood. Red cells and platelets may adhere and form clumps which vary in size between 15 and

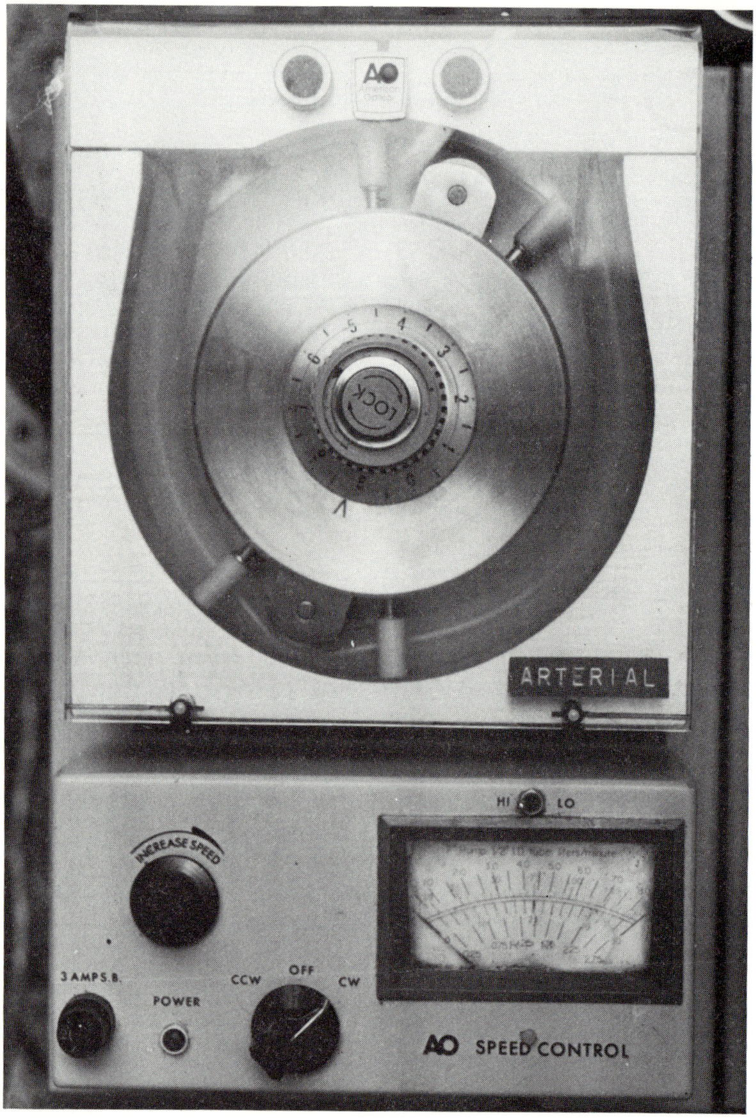

Figure 6.6
Roller pump. Tubing in device must be high quality silicone tubing.

200 μm. Embolization of these clumps to the tissues causes organ damage by small artery occlusion. All bypass circuits contain filters which remove the larger emboli, but in recent years much attention had been given to the effects and removal of the emboli of 15–40 μm in size. Many surgical teams now incorporate a 'microfilter' at some point in the circuit in an effort to remove these.

Non-pulsatile versus pulsatile flow

The flow from the roller pump is non-pulsatile and convincing evidence has been produced to show that this stimulates the renin–angiotensin system in the kidneys. Angiotensin is a potent vasoconstrictor and small vessel constriction is produced which temporarily or perhaps permanently impairs the functions of some organs.

If the pump flow can be made pulsatile, laboratory, biochemical and clinical evidence can be produced which shows a return to a more normal physiological situation. In spite of some doubts as to whether it is possible to provide truly pulsatile flow, there is a slow increase in the number of surgical teams using pulsatile flow, usually by means of a roller pump which is controlled by an acceleration–deceleration device.

Summary

Cardiopulmonary bypass is unphysiological and can be used only for relatively short periods. The surgery should be performed as quickly as possible so long as a complete and satisfactory repair or correction is performed. The problems arising from cardiopulmonary bypass are those of organ and tissue dysfunction, but the greater problem is created by inadequate removal of air from the left heart which is under direct surgical control and therefore largely preventable.

Persisting controversies

- Merits of pulsatile versus non-pulsatile flow.
- Bubble versus mebrane oxygenator and the indications for using each type.
- The ideal priming fluid.

Further reading

Gibbon, J.H. (1954) Application of a mechanical heart and lung apparatus to cardiac surgery. *Minn. Med.*, *37*, 171.

Gindoin, R., Laperche, Y., Martin, L., Awad, J. & Winchester, J. (1976) Disposable filters for microaggregate removal from extracorporeal circulation. *J. Thorac. Cardiovasc. Surg.*, *71*, 502.

Ionescu, M.I. (1981) *Techniques in Extracorporeal Circulation*, 2nd edn. London: Butterworths.

Kirklin, J.W, Du Shane, J.W., Patrick, R.T., Donald, D.E., Hetzel, P.S., Harshbarger, H.G. & Wood, C.H. (1955) Intracardiac surgery with the aid of a mechanical pump oxygenator (Gibbon type). Report of eight cases. *Proc. Staff Meet. Mayo Clin.*, *30*, 201.

Litwack, R.S., Jurado, J.A., Lukban, S.B., Mitchell, B.A., Kahn, M., Berger, S., Estioka, M.R. & Aledort, L. (1972) Perfusion without donor blood. *J. Thorac. Cardiovasc. Surg.*, *64*, 714.

Pacifico, A.D., Digerness, S. & Kirklin, J.W. (1970) Acute

alterations of body composition after open intra-cardiac operations. *Circulation*, *41*, 331.

Taylor, K.M., Wright, G.S., Reid, J.M., Bain, W.H., Caves, P.K. Walker, M.S. & Grant, J.K. (1978) Comparative studies of pulsatile and non-pulsatile flow during cardiopulmonary bypass, I and II. *J. Thorac. Cardiovasc. Surg.*, *75*, 569.

7 Complications of Surgery to the Valves of the Heart

Valve surgery produces some of the most spectacular benefits of cardiac surgery. All the evidence suggests that the operations cause an increase of life span, an improvement in the quality of that life and a relative freedom from complications. Nevertheless, cardiac valve surgery is very rarely curative. The nature of diseases causing the initial valvular disorder and the imperfect nature of valvular prostheses lead to the operations being palliative. Indeed, with the long-term survival of patients being so great, any individual having a valve operation is likely at some time in the future to have at least one more operation.

The ideal result of valve surgery is a patient who is able to function as well as his normal companions and live as long as they will. Objective examination of cardiac function should reveal normal haemodynamics and the operation should last as long as the patient lives. The usual result, however, is to change a patient with severe disease into a much less disabled patient with mild heart disease. The need for continuing medical and surgical care remains and many patients need to take cardiac drugs. The complications of valve surgery discussed here are listed in Table 7.1.

Failure to Recover Full Functional Capacity

The ability to exercise comfortably and live normally depends on many factors. Apart from the actual physical effects of the disease and the subsequent operation, it is important to appreciate that psychological and social factors play an enormous part in determining recovery (Table 7.2). Many patients have labelled themselves as cardiac cripples in the months and years before their operation and this will affect their perception of themselves afterwards in ways which are difficult to recognize and to change. Similarly, the attitudes and expectations of families and employers of such patients will have a major influence on the quality of recovery. There is an increasing awareness among those looking after such patients that too little attention has been paid to these factors in the past and that there should now be an extension of rehabilitation programmes in order to aid full recovery. Such programmes should be both physical and mental.

Table 7.1
Complications of valve surgery.

1	Failure to recover full functional capacity
2	Complications directly related to the valve operation itself
3	Complications of valvular prostheses

Table 7.2
Factors determining functional recovery after heart valve surgery.

1	Preoperative cardiac status
2	The quality of the valve operation
3	The quality of myocardial preservation
4	The presence of other diseases
	(a) Pulmonary vascular disease
	(b) Liver disease
	(c) Cerebral disease

Preoperative cardiac status

Valve disorders impose stresses on the heart and on associated organs such as the lungs and the whole body.

Valvular stenosis causes an obstruction to the passage of blood within the heart. As in any other obstruction, this causes a hypertrophy of the muscle upstream of that obstruction and effects due to poor flow downstream. Stenotic valves therefore lead to a poor cardiac output which causes tiredness and a marked inability to exercise. The hypertrophy of the muscle occurs as a result of the need to create excessive *pressures* in order to overcome the effects of the obstruction. The oxygen demands of the heart rise sharply and often outstrip the available supply. Consequently, symptoms due to valvular stenosis tend to occur sooner rather than later and to be severe. Indeed, many patients with stenosis come for surgery very early in the course of their disease. When surgery is successfully performed there is an immediate relief to the pressure burden and the heart begins to function better immediately.

Valvular regurgitation is quite different. The effect is to decrease the efficiency of the heart as a pump and the heart compensates by enlarging in order to pump increased *volumes*. This is a lesser insult than that imposed by an increased pressure load. In addition, the cardiac output can be maintained more easily. Consequently, valvular regurgitation tends to be well tolerated by the patient, but the burdens of regurgitation although of less immediate consequence to the heart, are equally damaging in the long term.

The result of these differences is that the patient with valvular stenosis develops symptoms early in the disease and presents much earlier for surgery, whereas the patient with valvular regurgitation has mild progressive symptoms for a number of years and tends to seek surgical operation much later. The effect on postoperative recovery is marked: operations for valve stenosis are less risky and carry better long-term recoveries than those for valvular regurgitation. However, no matter what the nature of the valve lesion, the degree of preoperative incapacity also has a major influence on the quality and length of postoperative survival. Those patients with cardiac symptoms at rest (New York Heart Association Class 4) do worse at every stage than comparable patients with symptoms of a lesser degree. Similarly, those patients with cardiac cachexia will do badly compared with patients of normal body weight.

The age of the patient is less important than might be imagined; although there is some impairment in short- and long-term recovery, some of the most impressive results of valve surgery are with elderly patients who have had operations for aortic stenosis.

Summary The length of illness before the operation and the nature of the valvular disorder are important determinants of postoperative survival and function. Impairment of function will be found in those patients referred to surgery late in the disease.

The quality of the valve operation

The normal human cardiac valve has remarkable hydraulic features. It opens at low pressures and closes quickly when needed. It permits large volumes of blood to flow through it without imposing obstruction. All of these features can be measured objectively at cardiac catheterization and it is extremely uncommon to find normal functioning in any valve which has been operated on or replaced. Consequently, what distinguishes a 'good' from a 'bad' operation is merely the degree of abnormality which remains.

Diseased valves may be suitable for valvotomy or repair. The operations preserve the existing valvular tissues. The merit of these conserving procedures is that the valve is durable and self repairing. The disadvantage is that the initial valvular disease remains and indeed, over the years, will progress. Most valve disorders in adults occur as a result of post-inflammatory scarring which is clearly progressive. Valvotomy will improve the pressure difference across the valve but will rarely bring this measurement back to the low or zero values of a normal valve. Similarly, a valve-conserving repair of regurgitation rarely gives the 100% competence of the normal valve.

Valve prostheses of whatever sort are even more abnormal. Not only are the haemodynamic imperfections more evident but also the materials are not self repairing. All valvular prostheses therefore have a finite and limited life span whether the prosthesis is made of man-made or animal materials.

Circumstances within the heart, such as the size of the valve ring and the chambers, will often lead to the substitution of a valve of an inappropriate size for that individual and so further decrease the quality of the valve operation. An 'imperfect' valvotomy may be judged as being superior to a valve replacement in an individual patient.

The quality of the valve operation clearly determines the capacity for functional recovery. However, it is not always completely under the surgeon's control since non-surgical factors may detract from the theoretical 'perfect' result. Clearly, sometimes technical and operative misjudgements will further diminish the quality of the valve operation and these are factors determined by the skill, experience and concentration of the surgeon.

The quality of myocardial preservation

If a satisfactory quality of valve operation is achieved and valvular function is improved at the end of the operation, the heart should function better than it did immediately before surgery. This is not always so and under these circumstances the myocardium has often been damaged during the operation. This damage may be permanent or temporary and it may not be avoidable. Nevertheless, the myocardial factor is an important determinant of postoperative function both in the short- and long-term and failure to preserve it must be counted as a complication of valvular surgery.

The essential function of the myocardium is to contract strongly in a co-ordinated manner. The energy-producing mechanisms within the myocardial cell therefore must be preserved. Since these are aerobic, the essence of myocardial preservation is to match the oxygen demands of the myocardium with oxygen availability and ensure an otherwise normal physiological milieu. This has been discussed in the section entitled 'Myocardial preservation' (see page 75). The difficulty of ensuring adequate myocardial protection in a diseased heart is greater than in a normal heart. Hypertrophy and fibrosis of the ventricular muscle often makes the adequacy of coronary blood flow and oxygen supply limited, and during cardiopulmonary bypass this inadequacy is increased. The coronary arteries may not be normal and obstructive lesions due to atheroma may further diminish the oxygen availability. Finally, various drugs and arrhythmias may increase oxygen demands.

To avoid myocardial damage is the main target of the surgeon during valve replacement. Before surgery, the state of the coronary arteries should be known by arteriography in all patients (except the young – say below 30 years) so that appropriate action can be taken if necessary. The heart rate and arterial pressure are controlled as described in order to preserve the ratio between demand and availability of oxygen. During the cardiopulmonary bypass, the surgeon has to choose between supplying the oxygen demands or using cardioplegia. At the time of writing, most surgeons use cardioplegia as the preferred method of intraoperative myocardial preservation (see Chapter 5).

The presence of other diseases

Certain valve disorders, notably those of the mitral valve, cause effects on other organs by a combination of increased back pressure and poor cardiac output. The lungs are particularly susceptible to venous hypertension and respond by undergoing an increase in wall thickness and reduction of the lumen in the smaller pulmonary vessels. Later, thrombosis of the small vessels may occur. These changes impair oxygen uptake and impede the flow of blood through the organ. Clearly, the changes will not resolve quickly, if at all, after mitral valve surgery and they may be so severe as to cause fatal low output syndrome. Certainly, the patient with pulmonary vascular disease will make a slow recovery after valve surgery and may take some years to reach maximal benefit.

In a similar manner, hepatic cirrhosis due to cardiac disorders will impede the chances of the patient having a complication-free operation and damage caused by cerebral emboli will obviously have the same effect.

Summary

The most serious complication of valvular heart surgery is failure to achieve a full functional recovery. Poor function is due to several factors. The preoperative cardiac status and the presence of other diseases are not under the surgeon's control, but the quality of the valve operation and the myocardial preservation are. Earlier referral for surgery will help to avoid this complication.

Careful assessment of ventricular function and of the coronary arteries will enable the surgeon to improve myocardial preservation. Preoperative investigation of valvular heart disease is rarely concerned with the diagnosis of the valvular lesion which is usually clinically evident or easily discernible with non-invasive tests such as ultrasound. The ventricular function and the coronary arteries are important risk factors meriting careful investigation.

Persisting controversies

- Timing of surgical referral, particularly in patients with valvular regurgitation.
- The methods of investigating patients with valvular heart disease before surgery.
- The methods of myocardial preservation.

Complications of Valve Operations

Closed mitral valvotomy

This operation is performed for pure mitral stenosis which has been shown to have non-calcified mobile cusps. The clinical signs of mobile cusps are an increased intensity of the first heart sound at the apex and the so-called 'opening snap' which occurs shortly after the second sound. Echocardiography is reliable in the diagnosis of mitral stenosis and can distinguish calcified and immobile cusps. Patients who have mitral regurgitation, other valve lesions or a history of arterial thromboembolism are unsuitable. If any doubt as to the mobility of the valve cusps or left atrial thrombus is present, the mitral valvotomy should be performed under 'open' conditions using cardiopulmonary bypass.

The operation is performed through a left anterior thoracotomy through the bed of the fifth rib. The lung is retracted posteriorly and the pericardium divided anterior to and parallel with the phrenic nerve. When the heart is exposed, examination will reveal a diastolic thrill over the left ventricle.

The left atrium is explored by inserting a finger in the left atrial appendage. Once the diagnosis is confirmed, an expanding dilator is passed through the apex of the left ventricle and guided through the narrowed orifice of the mitral valve. The dilator is then opened and the cusps which are adherent are split along the commissures thus relieving the stenosis.

Complications

Thromboembolism. The source of this is a thrombus in the left atrium and especially in the appendage. Introduction of the finger may dislodge the thrombus from this site. Therefore, before the appendage is clamped, its tip is amputated with a pair of scissors. Often a thrombus will be washed out in the gush of blood which ensues. The clamp should not be applied until a jet of fresh red blood has been seen. Once the clamp is applied, the finger is introduced and a thrombus may be felt in the main cavity of the left atrium. This is extremely dangerous and the operation should be abandoned as a closed procedure and performed using cardiopulmonary bypass. Once again, the exploring finger, in spite of favourable indications before operation, may find craggy calcium deposits in the valve cusps, especially in the commissures. To split such a valve would cause calcium emboli. As before, the operation needs converting into an open operation. The practice of proceeding in the presence of thrombus or calcium and temporarily occluding the carotids to prevent major cerebral embolism is unreliable and very little used.

Air embolism. It is very difficult to introduce air into the beating, filled heart. The only hazard here is that a bubble may be released when the dilator blades are separated. This hazard may be avoided by opening and closing the dilator under water a few times before it is inserted into the heart.

Bleeding. The apical wound to introduce the dilator is through the thick left ventricular muscle and rarely bleeds much. However, the left atrial appendage is friable and may tear. Tearing is often caused by too small a hole being made. The ideal size is one which will accommodate the proximal interphalangeal joint of the right index finger. After the finger is removed, the appendage is amputated and the stump repaired by a continuous everting stitch with over-and-over reinforcement.

Damage to the valve. Sometimes the dilator may tear a cusp – usually the anterior. The jet of regurgitation may be detected by the finger in the left atrium and always feels less than it actually is. Open repair or mitral valve replacement is indicated.

Inadequate valvotomy. After the dilator has been inserted and opened, it is withdrawn and the right index finger assesses the result. There is often a remaining length of commisural fusion and the finger or the dilator should be used to split this. Subsequently, it is important to feel the state of the subvalvular structures which may be causing obstruction. Digital pressure will often separate fusion at this point.

When the two cardiac incisions have been closed, the diastolic thrill over the left ventricle should have disappeared. The pericardium is loosely closed so as to prevent the lung adhering to the heart but not so tightly that tamponade may occur. The chest is closed with one basal drain.

After closed mitral valvotomy, most patients recover quickly. Any signs of low cardiac output or pulmonary oedema should raise the suspicion of an inadequate operation or of damage to the valve, and urgent investigation ordered.

Open mitral valve repair

These operations are performed using a median sternotomy and cardiopulmonary bypass which is obtained by bicaval cannulation removing blood and by aortic cannulation. When the circulation is supported by cardiopulmonary bypass, the ascending aorta is clamped and the cardioplegic solution run in under pressure.

The left atrium is opened from the right side. An incision is made in the epicardium overlying the atrial septum which lies just anteriorly to the right pulmonary veins. Sharp dissection enables the surgeon to pass 2 cm medially before opening into the posteriorly placed left atrium. The incision is then extended cephalad to the upper limit of the left atrium and caudad to the left atrium which lies behind the inferior vena cava. A retractor will then expose the mitral valve. The valvotomy or repair is then carried out under direct vision.

After repair, the competence of the valve needs to be tested. The usual way to do this is to fill the left ventricle with blood or fluid and look at how the valve appears. The conditions are of course highly artificial and therefore the test is extremely fallible.

Complications

Damage to the valve. This usually results from attempting to remove too much calcium or by dividing supporting chordae tendineae. Valve replacement is usually the only method of dealing with this.

Valve regurgitation may be due to one of three factors:

1 Dilated ring.
2 Stretched cusps.
3 Elongated or ruptured chordae.

A dilated ring may be reduced in size by using a prosthetic ring but other disorders will probably need valve replacement.

Failure to remove thrombus. The left atrial appendage should be inspected from within and any thrombus removed. Thrombus in the main cavity should be removed cleanly and in one piece by finding the plane of cleavage between it and the left atrial endocardium. Removal of left atrial thrombus by fragmentation is dangerous and to leave a shaggy, raw surface is to invite further formation of thrombus after the operation.

Air embolism is common after open mitral valve operations. The best method of prevention is to close the left atrial incision loosely with a continuous everting monofilament suture. The patient is then placed in a steep head-down position and as the heart is filled with blood and begins to contract, any air will escape through the loose suture line. As the shed blood fills up the pericardium and the suture line is submerged, the suture is tightened and haemostasis achieved. At this stage, it is possible to introduce the finger into the left atrium and detect any mitral regurgitation.

Mitral valve replacement

When the mitral valve is exposed, the surgeon may decide to replace it. Extensive disease and calcification of the valve, together with subvalvular disease are the usual indications for valve replacement.

Complications

Unsuitably prepared valve ring. The old valve should be excised to leave about 1 cm of cusp tissue in place. Calcification may sometimes make this impossible, particularly in the posterior ring. Removal of calcium is very hazardous if it extends into the valve ring and extreme care is needed to remove calcium precisely. If calcium is present in the valve ring posteriorly, it should be left for fear of causing atrioventricular disruption.

Unsuitable excision of subvalvular structures. The chordae should be excised just below the tip of the papillary muscles. If too long chordal stumps remain, they may engage the disc or ball of a mechanical valve and jam it. Too extensive an excision of papillary muscle may cause a hole in the left ventricular free wall.

Paravalvular leak (see below, page 136).

Disruption of the atrioventricular junction. This is the most dreaded operative complication of mitral valve replacement and is usually fatal. Its presence is diagnosed when bright red blood is seen coming from the left atrioventricular groove into the pericardium.

The causes are not precisely known, but the following factors are important:

1 Overexcision of calcification in the posterior mitral valve ring.
2 Suturing too deeply in this area.
3 Insertion of too large a valve prosthesis.
4 Undue elevation of the heart when the prosthesis is in place (as in removal of an apical left ventricular vent).

These factors should be avoided as treatment of the established disruption is virtually impossible. Those successes which have been recorded have been achieved by removal of the prosthesis and resewing the disruption from the inside.

Damage to the aortic valve. The aortic valve lies just anterior to the mitral valve and may be damaged by excessive dissection of the native mitral valve or by passing the sutures too deeply during valve replacement (Fig. 7.1).

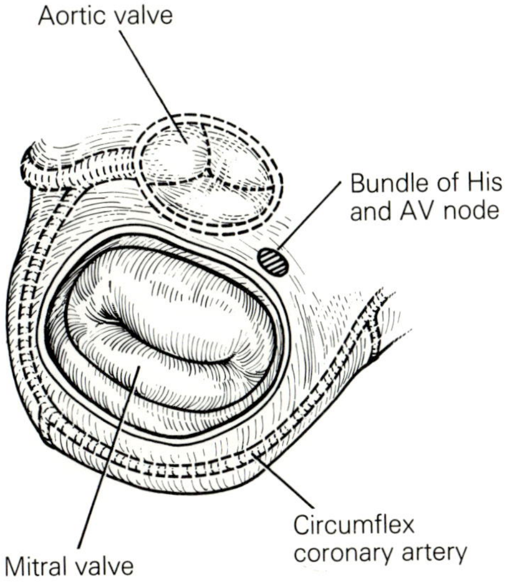

Figure 7.1 The anatomical relationships of the mitral valve.

Heart block. The atrioventricular node lies just medially to the medial commissure at the ring (Fig. 7.1) and may be damaged by a stitch placed too deeply at this point.

Aortic valve replacement

The diseases of the aortic valve which cause the need for valve replacement tend to cause some dilatation and thinning of the ascending aorta; this fact makes the operation easier to perform when replacing the valve itself but may cause problems with closure of the aorta.

After bypass is established, the left ventricle is decompressed by a suction vent placed in its apex and the ascending aorta is then clamped and opened. The aortic valve is excised and replaced with an appropriately sized prosthesis after a cardioplegic solution has been placed in each coronary orifice. The ascending aorta is then closed and the aortic clamp released. Air is evacuated from the left ventricle and a spontaneous circulation restarted.

Complications

Calcium embolism. Most diseased aortic valves are heavily calcified and difficult to remove as one piece. Many small pieces of calcium remain and are a potential hazard – not just to the brain but also to the heart. Prevention is achieved by removing the valve in one piece if possible. This is most easily done by cutting the diseased valve free with a sharp pointed scalpel as close to the aortic ring as possible where there is often a non-calcified plane. Any calcium remaining in the ring may be crushed and twisted free using Caldwell–Luc nasal sinus forceps. The danger of disruption of the valve ring is much less than in the case of the mitral valve.

Paravalvular leak (see below, page 136).

Bleeding after aortic valve replacement is most often from the aortic suture line. The aortic wall, although dilated, is very thin and great care has to be taken in closing the aortotomy. A fine (3/0 or 4/0) monofilament suture is placed in the usual manner, beginning at the right hand part of the incision. The first layer is an everting continuous horizontal mattress suture and this continues into a second continuous over-and-over suture which is then tied.

Any bleeding from the suture line is repaired using a horizontal mattress buttressed suture placed when the aortic pressure is low. On bypass, such a low pressure is achieved by reducing the pump flow to a very low level for a minute or so. After bypass, the aortic pressure may be safely lowered for a short time by placing a clamp across the inferior vena cava.

Tricuspid valve surgery

The tricuspid valve is operated on infrequently and it is usually possible to perform a repair. Replacement is only necessary when the subvalvular apparatus is diseased.

The major specific complication of tricuspid valve surgery is *complete heart block.* The bundle of His or the atrioventricular node are damaged by a stitch passing through the medial aspect of the valve. The diagram (Fig. 7.2) shows the structures within the atrial septum as seen from the right atrium. The ligament of Todaro may be identified by gentle traction on the medial lip of the coronary sinus.

All patients having valve surgery, but especially those having tricuspid procedures, are at risk from heart block. The routine insertion of a ventricular pacing wire is good practice. In most patients it will not be used and is removed on the seventh day after surgery, but in those patients who do develop heart block it is invaluable.

Complications of Valvular Prostheses

Two types of valve prosthesis are available:

1 Mechanical prostheses. These are made entirely of man-made material (Fig. 7.3).
2 Bioprostheses. These are partially or totally made of biological material – usually the aortic valve or pericardium. These bioprostheses are *not* grafts since the tissue has been killed and stabilized by a number of chemical treatments (Fig. 7.4).

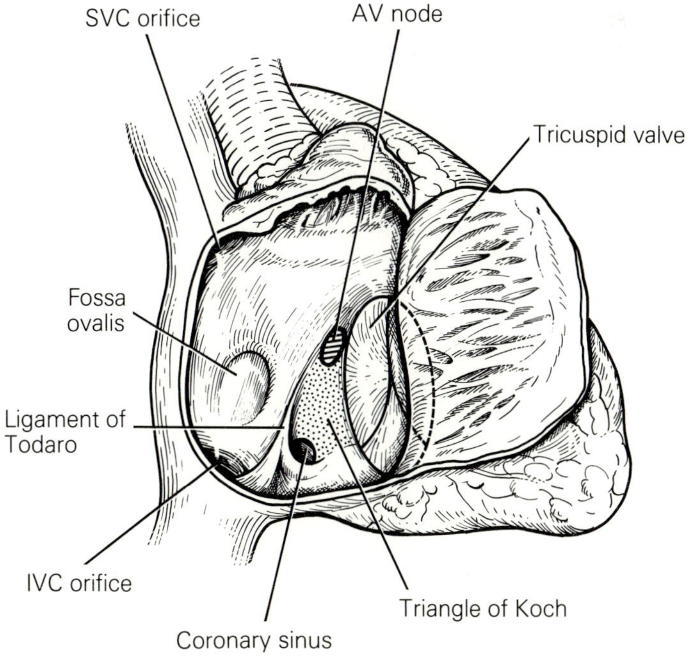

Figure 7.2 Location of the atrioventricular node within the right atrium.

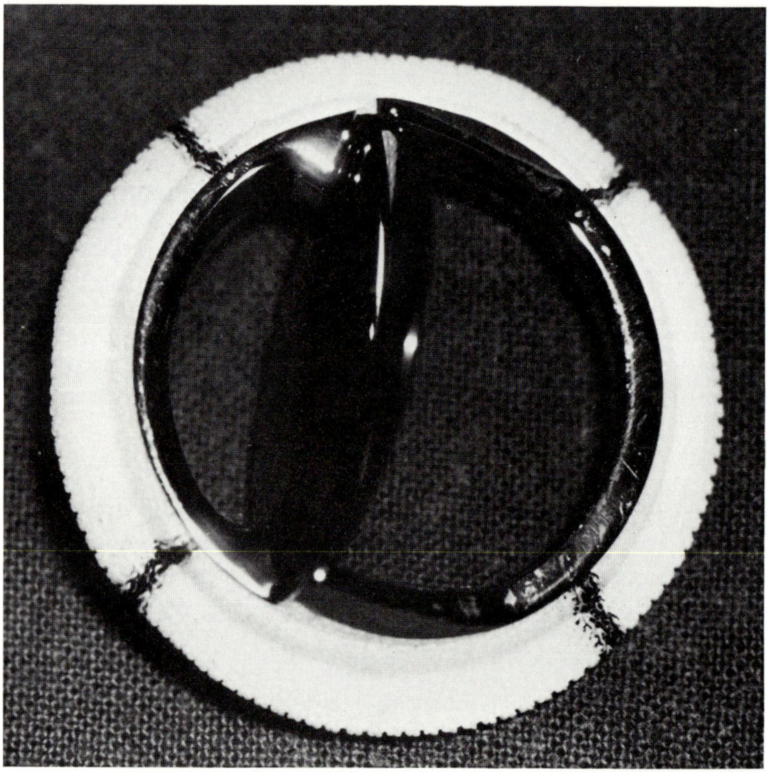

Figure 7.3
A commercially available 'tilting disc' mechanical valvular prosthesis.

Each type of valve has peculiar advantages, disadvantages and complications and these are listed in Table 7.3. It is inappropriate in this volume to discuss the choice of valve replacement and certainly no advice is given concerning the actual type of prostheses of the many commercially available. Each surgeon and patient will have preferences.

However, mechanical valves should never be used if long-term anticoagulation is a problem. Biological valves have been shown to degrade quickly in children, in patients with renal failure and in those with abnormal calcium metabolism.

Summary The ideal valve substitute does not exist. Each has specific advantages and disadvantages. To perform a valve replacement is to replace severe valve disease with lesser valve disease. The tendency to *sudden* failure of mechanical valves is, however, much less in biological valves.

Persisting controversies

- Choice between mechanical and biological valves.
- Requirement for anticoagulants in valve prostheses.

Disorders of function

The hydraulic performance of prosthetic valves is good, in that

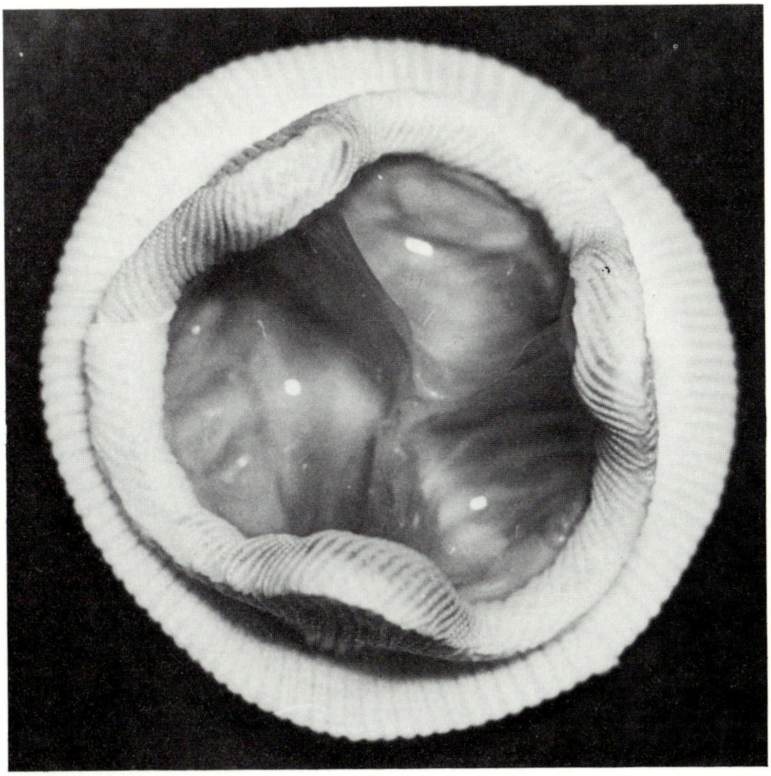

Figure 7.4
A commercially available porcine heterograft bioprosthesis.

Table 7.3
Characteristics of valve heart prostheses.

	Mechanical	*Biological*
Function	Good	Very good
Blood trauma risk	Moderate	Very low
Thromboembolism risk	High	Low
Need for anticoagulants	Always	Sometimes
Durability	Excellent	Unknown
Cost	High	High
Tendency to sudden failure	Present	Absent

they permit the passage of large volumes of blood with little obstruction and a very small amount of leakage is detectable when they are closed. Nevertheless, their performance never approaches the near perfection of the normal natural valve and, in addition, the pattern of the flow through the valve is usually qualitatively different. These imperfections constitute a form of mild valve disease and are acceptable only because they are a considerable improvement on the severe valve disease which has been removed.

The most severe stress for any valve is the ability to permit the high flows necessary during exercise without obstruction. The cardiac output during exercise may rise to 15–20 l/min with a stroke volume of perhaps 150 ml. This volume traverses the valve in about 200 msec. In a normal human valve there is a barely detectable pressure difference, but there is always a measurable pressure difference across a prosthetic valve. The size of this difference will depend on the type and size of prosthesis. The pressure difference becomes *clinically* important when it rises to 50 mmHg or more across an aortic valve prosthesis of 15 mmHg across a mitral prosthesis.

Prosthetic mechanical valves have a degree of regurgitation designed into their structure so as to produce a 'washing' effect which may reduce thrombosis. Biological valves have little regurgitation if any, but mechanical valves (especially tilting disc valves) permit regurgitation of about 4–8% of the forward volume to occur. This amount is clinically unimportant, but may produce murmurs which give rise to concern.

In general, biological valves perform somewhat better than the mechanical prostheses, except in their smaller sizes.

Summary Valvular prostheses have an impaired function compared with normal human valves and this must be accepted as an in-built complication. Larger valves tend to perform better than smaller and biological valves better than mechanical.

Blood trauma

The artificial character of the flow and the variable degree of obstruction posed by the valve may cause haemolysis which may be sufficiently severe to cause *clinical haemolytic anaemia*. This complication is almost always found with small mechanical valves in the aortic position and no treatment, apart from replacing the valve with a better one, is available. Most aortic mechanical prostheses will cause a certain amount of haemolysis which is detectable in the laboratory, but rarely becomes clinically significant.

Biological prostheses very rarely, if ever, cause haemolysis.

Thrombosis and thromboembolism

The foreign materials used in making both mechanical and biological prostheses lead to a tendency to induce thrombosis when they are inserted into the circulation (Fig. 7.5). This phenomenon will either derange the function of the valve, perhaps fatally, or lead to emboli which lodge in various organs. In order to prevent this complication, anticoagulants are given to patients starting about four days after the valve is inserted.

The tendency to thrombosis is determined by the design of the valve and the nature of the materials of which it is made. Most commercially available mechanical valves have a low tendency, as long as anticoagulants are given for life. Nevertheless, episodes of thrombosis or embolism will occur at a rate of 1–2% per patient year. There is therefore a significant risk of this

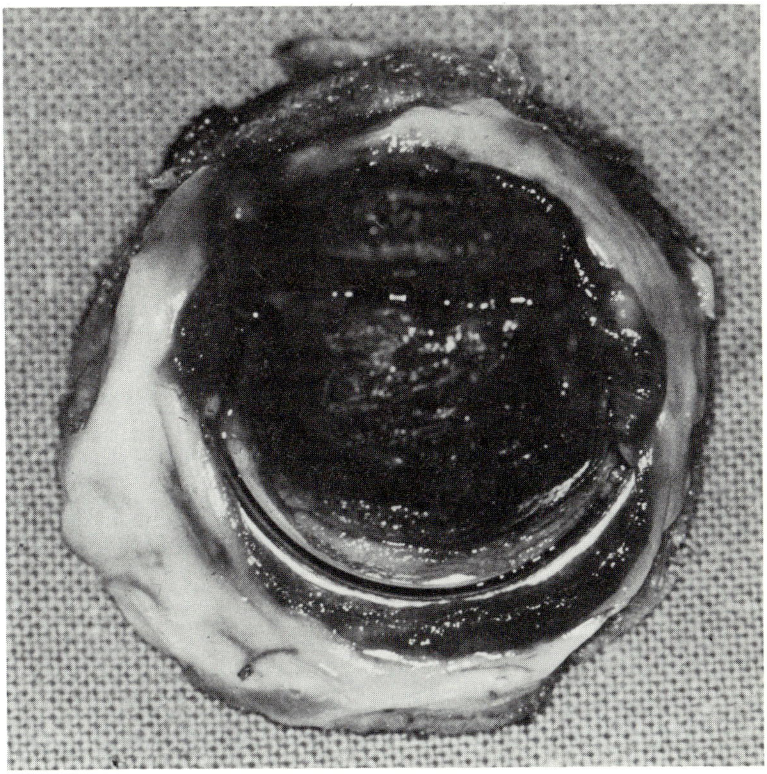

Figure 7.5
Thrombosed mechanical valvular prosthesis removed at emergency surgery four years after mitral valve replacement.

complication and it must be looked for in the follow up after valve insertion. Biological valves have a very low tendency to thrombosis and thromboembolism. Because of the man-made materials used in the sewing ring, it is usual to give anticoagulants for three months after biological valve replacement. Patients with atrial fibrillation should continue for life with anticoagulants because of the demonstrated benefits in preventing thrombosis and embolism in the paralysed atrium.

Anticoagulation is achieved by use of oral coumarin-type drugs such as warfarin. The dosage is controlled by testing the prothrombin time which should be prolonged to about twice normal. Once anticoagulants are started after mechanical valve replacement they should never be stopped, even if another surgical operation is performed. Most surgeons will find it difficult to detect any excess bleeding if the prothrombin time is maintained at about twice normal. Should anticoagulants be stopped and the prothrombin time reverts towards normal, the patient will be at a very high risk of thrombosis and embolism.

Thrombosis in a mechanical valve will lead to its failure which will kill the patient unless it happens sufficiently slowly for it to be recognized and treated. Massive thrombosis is often preceded by a slow build up of thrombosis around the valve orifice. Clinically, thrombosis should be suspected if a previously fit patient suddenly becomes incapacitated again. This may be reflected in a need for increasing diuretics or a change to a lighter job. Sudden severe pulmonary oedema and low cardiac output syndrome will clearly arouse suspicions of valve thrombosis.

Examination may be unrewarding apart from showing signs of obstruction. The valve clicks may become altered in their relative intensity to each other in early thrombosis and this difference may be heard with the stethoscope. Patients with early thrombosis may have a normal chest X-ray and electrocardiogram, but when obstruction occurs pulmonary oedema will be seen on an X-ray and the electrocardiogram will often show acute obstruction.

Early thrombosis of the valve is important to detect because valve replacement may avoid sudden catastrophes. Thus clinical suspicion should lead to full cardiac investigation, including pressure measurements, angiography and echocardiography.

Once the valve becomes massively thrombosed, the patient will die within a short time. There is therefore no time for investigation and valve replacement should be performed without delay. Most valves giving this complication are in the mitral position and are mechanical (see Fig. 7.5).

Embolism from thrombosis on a valve may cause a variable clinical picture. Most lodge in the brain, but the kidneys and the limbs are common sites. The picture may be obvious or very subtle and it is important at follow up to enquire about episodes of forgetfulness or disturbances of vision. Apart from making sure anticoagulation is adequately controlled, very little can be done about embolic episodes unless they are so frequent or damaging that the valve has to be replaced with one less prone to cause emboli. Cerebral emboli are the most dreaded complication of valve replacement and since fewer episodes occur with biological valves, most surgeons prefer to use these rather than mechanical valves.

Some emboli are composed of platelets and, if this can be proven, antiplatelet drugs such as aspirin may help.

Summary

All prosthetic valves have a tendency to induce thrombosis and thromboembolism and this can only be partially corrected by anticoagulants. Mechanical valves should be treated with anticoagulants for life, but biological valves may be suitable for a shorter period of anticoagulation, particularly if in the aortic position.

Thrombosis of a valve may begin slowly and sudden deterioration in a previously well patient should lead to suspicion of this. Acute massive thrombosis is a life-threatening event and needs urgent valve replacement.

Emboli are more common after mechanical valve insertions.

Persisting controversies

- The thrombotic tendencies of various mechanical and biological valves.
- The anticoagulant regimen.
- The early detection of thrombosis on a valve.
- The place of antiplatelet drugs given in conjunction with anticoagulants.

Durability

Normal cardiac valves are self repairing. The stresses acting on them cause minute areas of damage which heal. Prosthetic valves do not have this ability and consequently will ultimately wear out. A prosthetic valve will open and close some 40 million times each year and must be manufactured extremely precisely in order to prevent early mechanical failure. Inevitably, in a large number of valves, there will be a certain small percentage which fail at the outset and such attrition will continue over the years that follow. It is impossible to talk about an *average* survival for a valve. Its durability can only be assessed in vivo by the construction of an actuarial survival curve which accurately reflects the yearly depletion of the whole group.

Mechanical prosthetic valves are extremely durable both in vitro and in vivo. Although an earlier generation of mechanical valves often failed because of biological problems when implanted, today's valves made of man-made material are the product of experience thus gained and have a very low attrition rate.

The durability of biological valves is much more doubtful but what is known suggests that a maximum life of 10–15 years is to be expected. Extensive experience in the implantation of homograft valves suggests this, but methods of preparation have since changed and these will clearly influence longevity. A low rate of deterioration is only found in the first few years after implantation and subsequently the rate begins to accelerate. Degradation of a biological valve is rapid in those patients who are young or who have renal failure or any other abnormality of calcium metabolism.

The worn-out valve is recognized by the development of insufficiency or perhaps obstruction. Unless thrombosis supervenes, as it may well do on a damaged surface, this will be a slow process, and investigation and prosthetic replacement can be carried out before severe clinical deterioration occurs.

Summary Durability is an important consideration in prosthetic valve choice. Mechanical valves have a high durability. Biological prostheses are less durable over a period of several years.

Conclusion

There is no perfect cardiac valve substitute. Mechanical prostheses are durable but have an impaired function and an increased tendency to thrombose compared with biological prostheses. Biological prostheses work well, but will probably need replacement much sooner than the mechanical valves. The choice of valve prosthesis will depend on the individual preferences of the patient and surgeon. The ultimate feature which has to be considered, however, is the tendency to sudden failure. This is higher in mechanical than biological valves where failure tends to occur relatively slowly, permitting solutions to be found.

Persisting controversies

- Choice of mechanical or biological cardiac valve prosthesis.
- Methods of improving durability.
- Agreement on a standard protocol for comparing different valves to allow rational choices to be made.

Prosthetic Valve Endocarditis (PVE)

Bacterial contamination is dealt with extremely efficiently in the human and only rarely does infection occur. There are four situations, however, where contamination very easily becomes infection and these are:

1 Virulent organisms.
2 Reduced immunity.
3 The presence of a foreign body.
4 The presence of a pathological 'space'.

A prosthetic heart valve is a foreign body and its implantation will encourage contamination to become sepsis.

In the published literature, between 1 and 3% of all cardiac valves implanted will become infected and about one-half of these patients will die as a result. Prosthetic valve endocarditis is a major complication of valve replacement.

Bacteriology

The valve becomes the seat of infection for a wide variety of organisms. These vary from virulent pathogens such as *Staphylococcus aureus* and pseudomonal organisms to those which are non-pathogenic except in the presence of a foreign body such as *S. epidermidis* and diphtheroid organisms. The contamination usually occurs in the perioperative period and the period of highest risk is during the operation. The time spent in intensive care is also important, particularly if the body's defences are temporarily reduced as a result of low output syndrome. If the infection is caused by 'pathogens', it will become obvious in the first few days or weeks after surgery; if the infecting organism is a normal 'non-pathogen', the low grade infection may not declare itself for up to a year after the operation.

Much less commonly, prosthetic valve endocarditis (PVE) may result from bacteraemias caused by other conditions such as dental abscesses or diverticulitis.

Pathology

The infection causes vegetations to form on the prosthetic valve. These may embolize at any stage. Vegetation and abscess formation may occur between the sewing ring of the valve and the patient's tissues. This process will threaten the suturing of the valve which holds it in place and may give rise to a large abscess extending into other parts of the heart such as the interventricular septum (Fig. 7.6). Sudden valve failure and regurgitation may occur (Fig. 7.7).

Clinical picture

The patient often has a complicated postoperative course. Depending on the nature of the infecting organism, at some time after the operation the patient will become unwell and possibly develop clinical or radiological cardiac failure. Examination will show a pyrexia which may be quite slight. The valve may be functioning normally in the early stages. Splinter haemorrhages may suddenly appear in the nail beds. Sudden and catastrophic deterioration may occur at any time.

Investigation

The patient is usually anaemic and there may be a polymorphonuclear leucocytosis. Multiple (10+) blood cultures should be sent in the first 24 hours. If positive, they will indicate the nature of the organism and its bacteriological sensitivities. Sometimes, however, no positive result is obtained. The urine

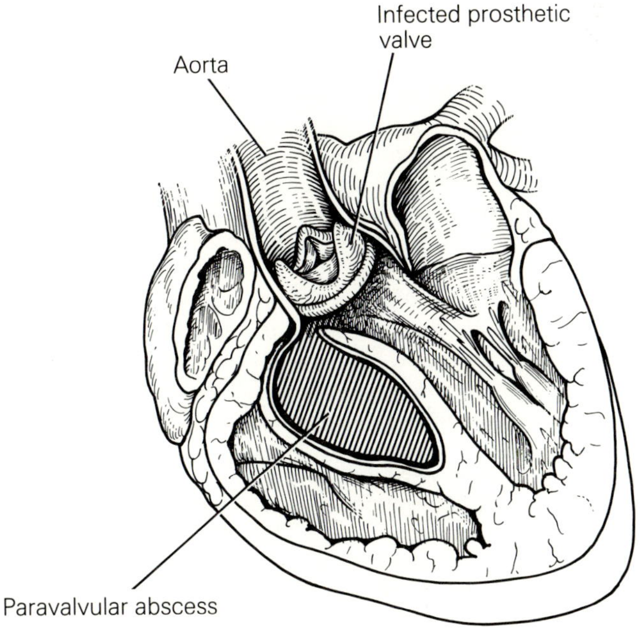

Figure 7.6 Paravalvular abscess extending into the interventricular septum.

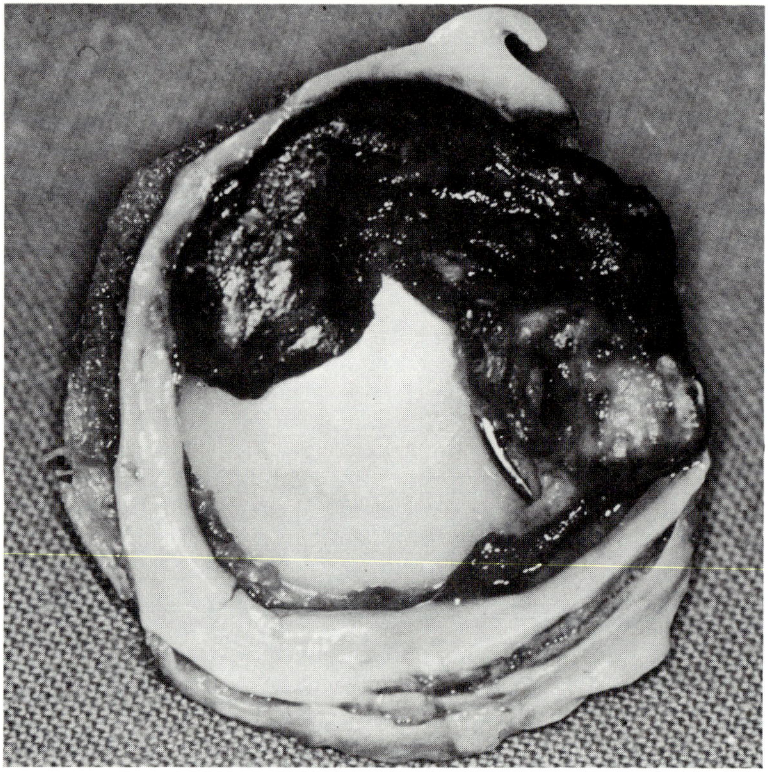

Figure 7.7 Infected valve prosthesis. The vegetation shown caused acute regurgitation.

and sputum should be examined because infection in the lungs or kidneys may produce a very similar clinical picture.

Differential diagnosis
The early diagnosis of PVE is extremely difficult, and often the decision has to be made on rather sparse and conflicting evidence. The cardinal and specific diagnostic test is the blood culture, but regrettably blood cultures are not totally sensitive.

Apart from infection in other systems, the only other major mimic of PVE is the postcardiotomy syndrome. This syndrome occurs after cardiac surgery and is due to either an autoimmune phenomenon or a low grade viral infection. It causes malaise and pyrexia. There is usually a high erythrocyte sedimentation rate and lymphocytosis. Blood cultures are negative. The syndrome rapidly resolves with aspirin or steroid treatment.

Prevention of PVE
1 All patients having cardiac surgery should have antibiotic prophylaxis. The type of drugs used will depend on local circumstances. Certain points are agreed:
(a) the prophylaxis must begin just before the surgical operation;

(b) prophylaxis should continue for at least five days;
(c) the narrowest spectrum of antibacterial activity should be used in order to prevent superadded infection.

2 The skin should be prepared before surgery. An electric razor should be used to prevent minor abrasions. The patient should take a bath in an extremely dilute povidone-iodine solution. In the operating theatre, at least five minutes should be spent scrubbing the skin with an antiseptic solution.

3 Contamination in the operating theatre can be reduced by an expeditious operation carried out by laconic surgeons with as few people present as possible. These conditions do not provide ideal circumstances in which to teach and some modification may be necessary.

4 All catheters, probes and injections should be given in an aseptic manner, not only in the operating theatre but also in the intensive care ward. Early removal of endotracheal tubes, drips and indwelling cannulas is desirable.

5 After the patient is discharged, acute infective illnesses and dental treatment, especially scaling, should be covered by antibiotics.

Treatment of PVE

Once the diagnosis is made, intravenous administration of high dose antibiotics is started. Ideally, this should be done in consultation with a bacteriologist. If a positive blood culture shows a specific organism, the appropriate antibiotics are given. If no positive cultures are obtained, the types of antibiotics used will depend very much on local circumstances and practice. Our practice has been to use gentamicin under these circumstances. If there is complete resolution of pyrexia and the patient feels better within 48 hours, the treatment should be continued for six weeks.

Evidence of cardiac failure due to valve dysfunction or arrhythmia leads to urgent surgery. Similarly, if the pyrexia has not completely resolved in 48 hours, the likelihood of a satisfactory outcome is very low. Valve replacement should be planned at this early stage rather than waiting for the patient to become toxic and jaundiced and in cardiac failure, often with large abscesses in the natural valve ring. Often at the second operation, the reasons for failure to respond to antibiotic treatment alone will be found. A paravalvular abscess is a common finding (see Fig. 7.6) and often the valve is unduly loose in its seating.

Not everyone agrees with this surgical approach to PVE preferring instead a much longer course of antibiotics. The mortality rate of PVE is high and, once failure to respond to antibiotics is demonstrated, we believe the valve should be replaced.

Summary

PVE is a dangerous complication of valve replacement. The

infection is usually caused at surgery and may be very indolent, declaring itself up to a year after operation.

The infecting organisms may be those normally found on the skin and termed 'non-pathogens'. The diagnosis may be easy, if positive blood cultures are obtained, or very difficult. Early vigorous treatment with antibiotics should be started and urgent surgery performed, unless a rapid resolution of the infection occurs.

Conclusion

Prosthetic valve endocarditis must be regarded as a late complication of the surgical operation which is largely preventable. The presence of a foreign body within the circulation poses grave dangers from both infection and valve dysfunctions. Antibiotics may be expected to be only partially successful in the treatment of PVE and removal of the infected foreign body may be the only effective form of treatment.

Persisting controversies

- Timing and place of surgery in PVE.
- Antibiotic prophylaxis.
- Diagnosis of PVE in the absence of positive blood cultures.

Paravalvular Leak

This complication is not strictly related to the valve prosthesis itself but to the manner of its insertion into the patient's heart. Valve prostheses have to be stitched into the native valve ring after removal of the diseased natural valve, and the sutures alone are responsible for holding the valve in position indefinitely because the prosthesis does not become firmly incorporated into the tissues of the valve ring. Consequently a leak may occur between the prosthetic ring and the natural ring and will give rise to regurgitation. Depending on the size of the leak, there will be variable symptoms and signs, and perhaps impairment of cardiac function.

Causes of paravalvular leak

1 Inadequate surgical technique.
2 Unsuitable prosthetic sewing ring.
3 Poor quality native valve ring.
4 Prosthetic valve endocarditis.

The most important factor causing paravalvular regurgitation is the manner in which the prosthesis is sewn into the heart. A satisfactory technique will accommodate to and overcome problems of a weak native valve ring or an unsuitable prosthetic sewing ring.

The suture material should be unabsorbable and strong – most surgeons prefer 00 size. The sutures must pass into the fibrous annulus of the valve, but not so deeply as to injure underlying structures. Interrupted sutures give a sounder suture line than continuous (Fig. 7.8). If the native valve ring is weak, multiple interrupted sutures are inserted in a horizontal, mattress fashion and each is buttressed by a pledget of Dacron felt (Fig. 7.9). As the valve is lowered into position, each suture is tied at least six times to prevent it becoming loose.

Sometimes the native annulus is so weakened by disease that the insertion of a valve becomes very difficult. The mitral valve annulus may become so diseased as to make satisfactory insertion virtually impossible. There are important underlying structures, such as the circumflex coronary artery, lying deep to the annulus at all points and deep insertion of suture is very dangerous. In the case of aortic valve replacement, careful dissection of the aortic root will allow sutures to be passed through the aortic ring and wall and then buttressed externally (Fig. 7.10).

Recognition of paravalvular regurgitation

The ease of diagnosis depends on the size of the paravalvular leak. Small leaks, due to say disruption of one stitch, are insignificant from the haemodynamic point of view and may often not give rise to an audible murmur. At the other end of the

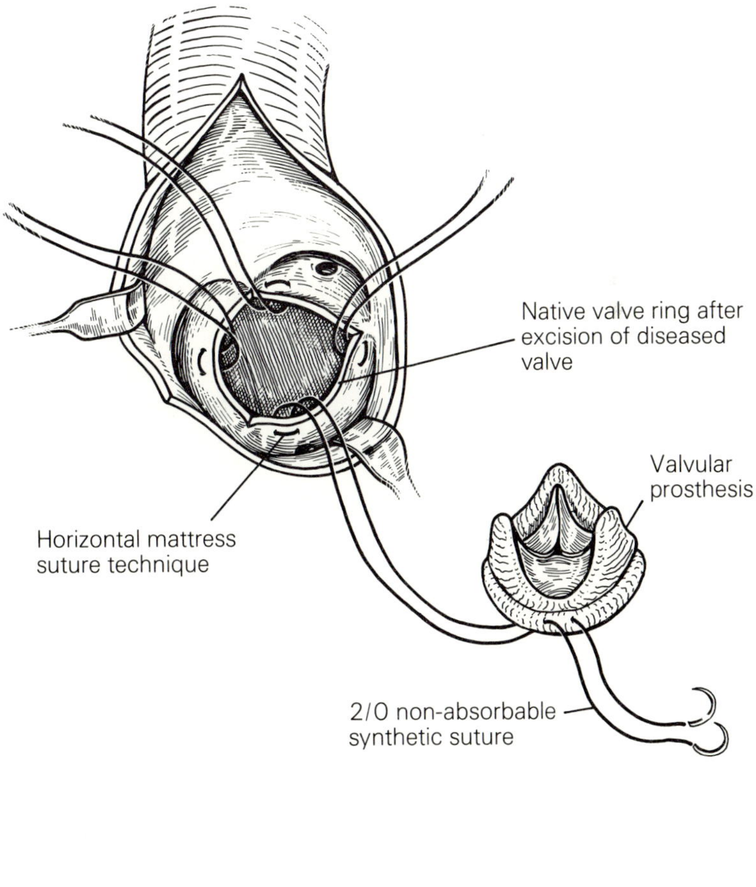

Figure 7.8
Suture technique in one method of valve insertion.

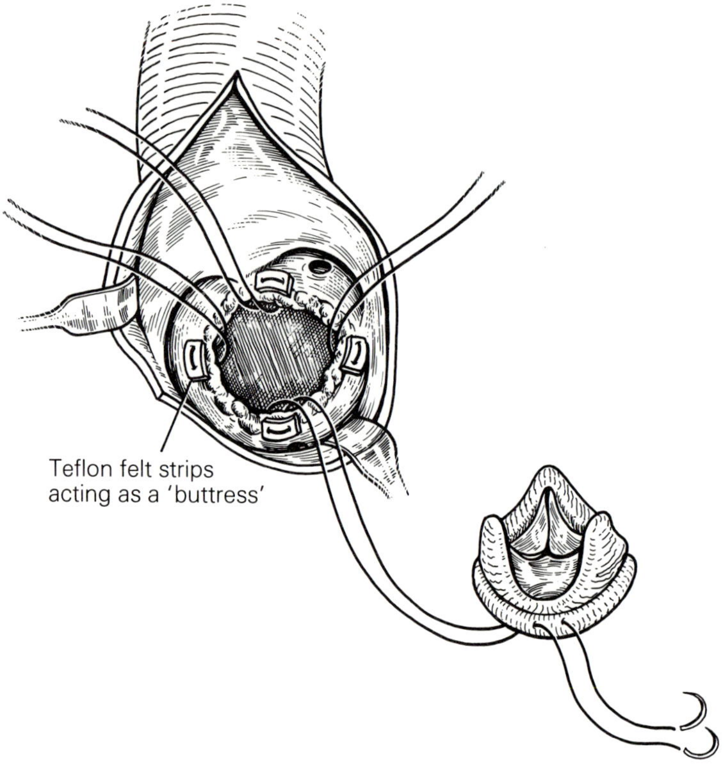

Figure 7.9
Alternative method of valve insertion if the native ring is diseased or friable.

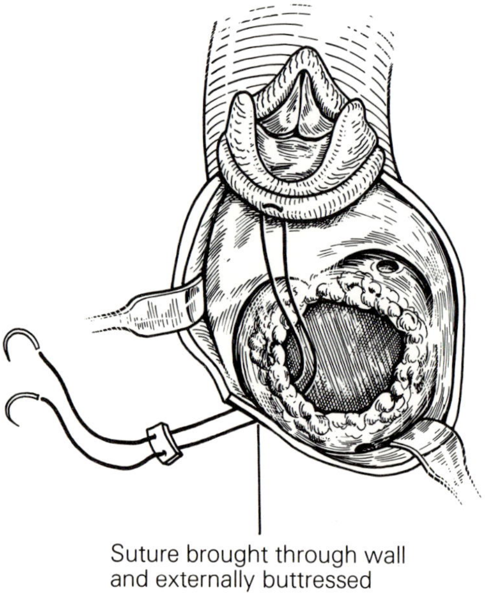

Figure 7.10
Another method of aortic valve insertion useful if the native ring is virtually destroyed by the disease process (as in endocarditis).

scale, disruption of a large length of the suture line will give rise to such massive regurgitation that low cardiac output and cardiac failure are caused.

In very large paravalvular leaks there may be no murmur, particularly if the mitral valve is affected. Such large leaks occur in the immediate postoperative period and the severe effects can only be treated by further open-heart surgery. Paravalvular regurgitation of this degree in the aortic valve is very rare and usually gives an audible diastolic murmur as well as a collapsing pulse.

Most patients will have a smaller paravalvular leak which impairs their ultimate recovery and this problem must be considered in every patient who has a disappointing result to valvular heart surgery. Clinical evidence of a murmur is valuable in the case of aortic valve replacements but very misleading after mitral valve replacement. Left ventricular angiography is the most reliable way of showing a mitral paravalvular leak. Whether or not such paravalvular leaks are repaired depends on the effects caused on the haemodynamic status of the patient and whether the turbulence of the leak causes haemolysis.

Correction of a paravalvular leak requires further open-heart surgery. The temptation merely to repair the leak is very strong, but often a strong repair can only be achieved by replacement of the valvular prosthesis.

Disruption of the valve ring

This is a rare but usually fatal complication of valve replacement. It is caused by:

1 Forcible insertion of too large a prosthesis.
2 Distortion of the natural valve ring.
3 Disease in the natural valve ring.

Treatment of disruption of the valve ring is virtually impossible in the mitral valve, but feasible with difficulty in the aortic, and so prevention must be given priority of attention.

The valve prosthesis must be carefully sized before insertion. The surgeon always wishes to insert the largest prosthesis possible but too large a prosthesis will distort and strain the natural valve ring, leading to a tendency to rupture. Therefore, in sizing the valve ring, the correct valve size will be the largest obturator which will pass freely. In those patients having mitral and aortic valve replacements, the sizing of the aortic valve replacement must be done after mitral valve replacement is completed because of the distortion which inevitably occurs.

The natural valve ring may disrupt after valve replacement if the heart is distorted. This is particularly liable to occur after mitral valve replacement when the apex of the left ventricle is elevated to remove air. Some other means of removing air from the left ventricle should be used.

Most ring disruptions occur in the mitral valve area and are due to disease in the ring leading to thinning of the atrioventricular tissues. Obviously very little can be done about this condition, but the tendency to disruption can be minimized by avoiding distortion of the heart in removing air.

Recognition of ring disruption

Recognition of ring disruption is all too easy. Bright red blood will be seen externally over the valve ring when the heart is supporting the circulation. In some cases the leak is so slight that it is not recognized and only later, when a false aneurysm is discovered, is the situation revealed. In most cases, the bleeding is so severe that it must be dealt with during the operation.

Treatment of valve disruption

Attempts at external repair are ineffective in the case of mitral disruption but may work in aortic. Usually the prosthesis will need removing and a new one inserted using multiple, deep, buttressed sutures. Even if external repair is attempted, cardiopulmonary bypass and the subsequent control of blood pressure is essential.

Summary

Valve ring disruption after valve replacement is extremely difficult to treat and great attention is given to its prevention. Avoidance of too large a prosthesis and of distorting the heart will reduce the incidence of disruption.

Persisting controversies

- Technique of removing air after valve replacement.
- Most effective way of repairing valve ring disruption.

Air Embolism

This is discussed on page 103 but no apology is made for repeating two points about this, the most common complication of heart surgery. The left atrium and ventricle are usually commodious and hypertrophied in left-sided valvular heart disease and air is easily trapped in either chamber. In addition, the insertion of a rigid valve creates new artificial regions in which air may be trapped.

Late Complications of Valvular Prostheses

The late complications of valvular prostheses occur at any time after the first year following surgery. Many are related to the valve simply wearing out (as already pointed out, a prosthesis is required to open and close some 40 million times a year) or to the body's response to the valve.

Causes (Table 7.4)
All of these causes lead to *valve dysfunction*.

Table 7.4
Causes of late valve complications.

1 Wear of the components of the prosthesis
2 Thrombosis
3 Tissue overgrowth
4 Calcification of biological valves

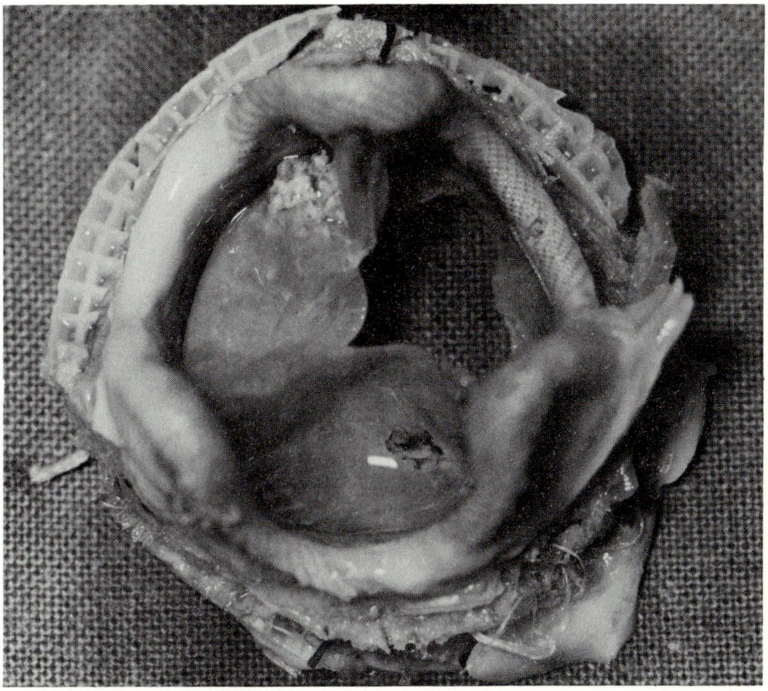

Figure 7.11
A 'worn-out' bioprosthesis which had been inserted five years before.

Wear of the components of the prosthesis

The durability of individual parts of the valve will depend on the stresses those parts suffer. The leaflets of a biological valve will wear at the part which undergoes most flexion (Fig. 7.11). The cage of a ball valve (e.g. Starr Edwards) will wear at its apex where the ball is stopped on each excursion (Figs 7.12, 7.13). The effects may be very variable – a slow worsening of valvular function or perhaps an increasing rate of haemolysis.

Thrombosis

This complication affects mainly, but not exclusively, mechanical prostheses. As stated previously, anticoagulants are given to all patients with mechanical prostheses in an effort to prevent this complication. Although poor anticoagulant control will dispose the patient to thrombosis, it may also occur without warning even in those whose anticoagulant control has been perfect for many years. Such catastrophic events nearly always affect the mitral rather than the aortic valve.

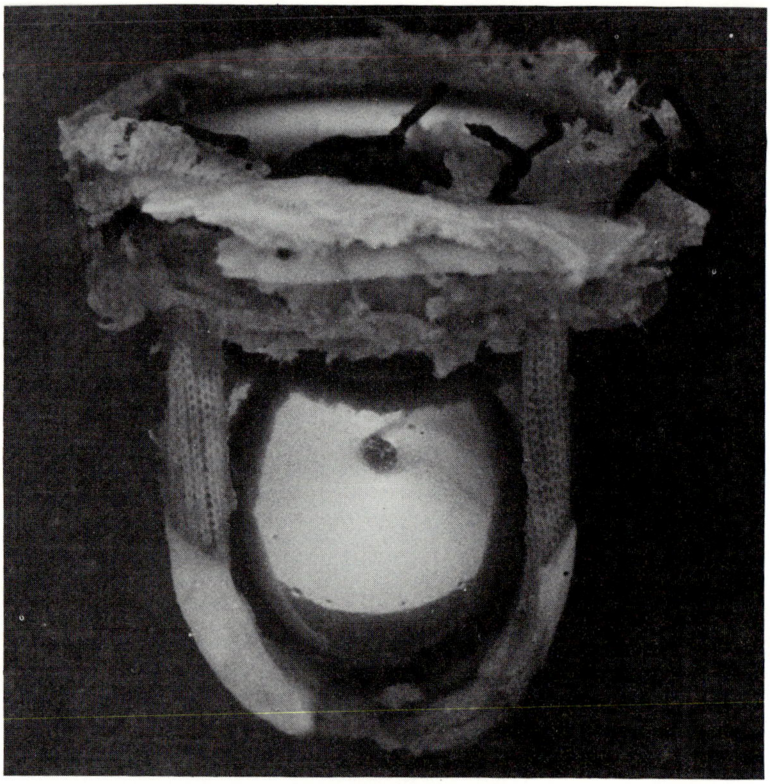

Figure 7.12
Wear of a mechanical ball valve.

Tissue overgrowth

The implantation of the prosthesis is followed by the deposition of fibrin on the fabric covered parts of the valve, such as the sewing ring. As time passes, organization of this fibrin occurs and results in a fibrous covering to the fabric. This is usually thin and does not encroach on the orifice of the valve. For reasons which are imperfectly understood, the fibrous tissue may become much thicker and extend to limit the orifice of the valve, producing an effective valvular stenosis or preventing full closure of a mechanical valve.

Calcification of biological valves

Calcification of any implanted biological tissue will always occur given time and this is true of biological valvular prostheses. There is ample evidence to show that microscopic calcification is seen within a few months of implantation and is progressive. In young patients or those with terminal renal failure, the process is very rapid. The cusps become effectively stenotic and may rupture. In otherwise healthy adults, most biological valves will be expected to calcify and fail after about ten years, but there is a wide individual variation.

Detection of late complications of valvular prostheses

The usual clinical picture is that of a patient who has had several

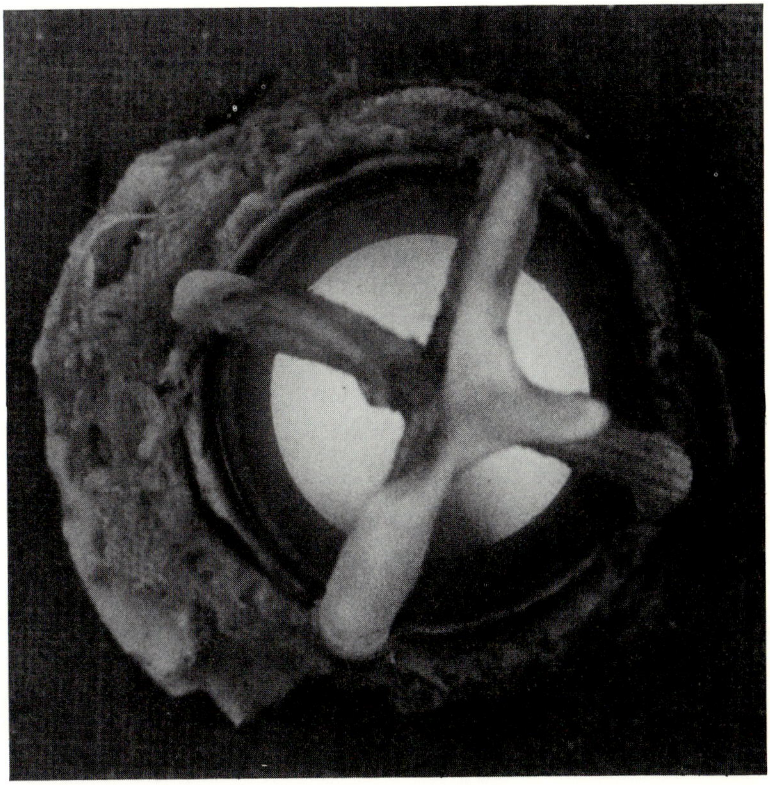

Figure 7.13
Tearing of the cloth over the struts of a mechanical ball valve.

years of well-being and good cardiac function after valve replacement showing again the symptoms and signs which led him to seek surgery in the first place. This is clearly distinct from the patient who has never had a good result with valvular surgery, whether it be due to myocardial damage suffered at the time of operation, other disease or an imperfect valve prosthesis.

The importance of following up patients after valve replacement is to detect such patients as soon as possible after they begin to deteriorate. Early investigation should be performed and whatever steps taken to remedy the valvular problem – usually by second operation. The doctors looking after such follow up must therefore be alert to the problem and when detected, the problem should not be ameliorated by changes in drug treatment such as an increase in the dose of diuretics. Such measures waste time and may merely make the final valve failure less easy to manage.

Since the performance characteristics of many valves in vivo are unknown, truly objective documentation may be difficult to obtain. However, if investigation of the patient shows that ventricular function is good and the coronary arteries normal, the suspicion of valve dysfunction must be very strong. In the end, a fruitless surgical exploration is preferable to leaving a patient to die with a malfunctioning prosthesis.

Summary
The prosthetic cardiac valve may show wear thrombosis, tissue overgrowth or calcification, leading to valve dysfunction. A characterisitc clinical history is obtained and should lead to early investigation and, if necessary, a further valve replacement. The investigation of such patients by cardiac catheterization and non-invasive means may be misleading. The temptation to manipulate the drugs which a patient is taking should be resisted until the nature of the problem has been resolved.

Persisting controversies
- The objective documentation of valve dysfunction.
- The role of early surgery and further valve replacement.

Anticoagulants and Valve Replacement

As stated above, anticoagulants are given to patients who have had valve replacements for two reasons, prevention of thrombosis and prevention of embolism (see page 129). All patients after valve replacement of any kind start on oral anticoagulants four days after surgery. The drug most commonly used is warfarin and a rather lower initial dose (4 mg) is used. The dosage is controlled by frequent estimations of the prothrombin time. After three months, those patients with biological valves who are in sinus rhythm may stop anticoagulants but all others should continue indefinitely.

Several problems arise from the need for long-term anticoagulants. These problems are:

1 Bleeding tendency.
2 Interaction of warfarin with other drugs.
3 The need for other surgical operations.

Bleeding tendency
Such a tendency in the anticoagulant patient may produce nose bleeds or haematuria. When episodes occur, the prothrombin time should be checked. If the prothrombin time is elevated, it is preferable to omit some doses of warfarin rather than to give vitamin K by injection since the latter may bring the clotting mechanisms of the patient abruptly back to normal and cause thrombosis of the valve. A patient with a peptic ulcer presents difficult problems and may need a biological valve for the reasons given above.

Drug interaction
Many drugs will alter the effect of warfarin on the prothrombin

time and the dosage of warfarin will need to be adjusted accordingly. Various antibiotics (especially broad-spectrum agents) and drugs used in the treatment of epilepsy displace warfarin from its binding to serum proteins and alter its coagulant effect. When other drugs are given to a patient on warfarin, the possibility of altering its action must be considered.

Need for other surgical operations

With a patient on warfarin after valve replacement, the greatest danger of thrombosis or embolism occurs when the issue of anticoagulant control arises if the patient needs to undergo other surgery. The inclination of the operating surgeon and the anaesthetist is to stop warfarin and give vitamin K. This is very dangerous and may lead to the patient's death from massive valve thrombosis. The correct strategy is to persuade the surgeon that he should perform surgery with the prothrombin time at 1.5–2.0. Afterwards most surgeons report that it was difficult to detect any unusual bleeding and complications very rarely occur. The practice of stopping oral anticoagulants and giving heparin gives the worst conditions possible for both patient and surgeon.

Finally, there are some patients in whom anticoagulant therapy should be cut short or never started. Those patients with active peptic ulceration arising in the postoperative period are obviously at risk from bleeding if anticoagulated. If such a patient has a biological aortic valve replacement, the risks of omitting anticoagulants altogether are less than the risks of giving them.

The present generation of biological prostheses, in particular, have very low thrombotic tendencies and if doubt over the safety of anticoagulant therapy arises, these are the prostheses of choice.

Further reading

Applebaum, A., Kouchoukos, N.T., Blackstone, E.H. & Kirklin, J.W (1976) The early risks of mitral valve surgery. *Am. J. Cardiol.*, *37*, 201.

Belcher, J.R. & Somerville, W. (1955) Systemic embolism and left auricular thrombosis in relation to mitral valvotomy. *Br. Med. J.*, *2*, 1000.

Boyle, D., MacDonald, L., Resnekov, L. & Ross, D.N. (1966) Experience with bypass surgery in coronary arterial disease complicating aortic valvular disease. *Br. Heart J.*, *28*, 428.

Braunwald, C., Braunwald, N.S., Ross, J., Jr & Morrow, A.G. (1965) Effects of mitral valve replacement on pulmonary vascular dynamics of patients with pulmonary hypertension. *N. Engl. J. Med.*, *273*, 509.

Cohn, L.H. & Gallucci, V. (ed.) (1982) *Cardiac Bioprostheses*. New York: York Medical Books.

Herr, R., Starr, A., McCord, C.W. & Wood, J.A. (1965) Special problems following valve replacement. *Ann. Thorac. Surg.*, *i*, 403.

Hyler, J.C. (1972) Mechanical malfunction and thrombosis of prosthetic heart valves. *Am. J. Cardiol.*, *30*, 396.

Linhart, J.W. & Wheat, M.W., Jr (1967) Myocardial dysfunction following aortic valve replacement. The significance of coronary artery disease. *J. Thorac. Cardiovasc. Surg.*, *54*, 259.

Magilligan, D.J., Lewis, J.W., Fara, F.M., Lee, M.W., Alam, M., Riddle, J.M. & Stein, P.D. (1980) Spontaneous degeneration of porcine bioprosthetic valves. *Ann. Thorac. Surg.*, *30*, 259.

Oyer, P.E., Stinson, E.B., Griepp, R.B. & Shumway, N.E. (1977) Valve replacement with the Starr Edwards and Hancock prostheses; comparative analysis of late morbidity and mortality. *Ann. Surg.*, *186*, 301.

Silver, M.M., Pollock, J., Silver, M.D., Williams, W.G. & Trusler, G.A. (1980) Calcification in porcine heterografts in children. *Am. J. Cardiol.*, *45*, 685.

Teply, J.F., Grunkemeier, F.L., Sutherland, H.D., Lambert, L.E., Johnson, V.A. & Starr, A. (1981) The ultimate prognosis after valve replacement; an assessment at 20 years. *Ann. Thorac. Surg.*, *32*, 111.

8 Complications of Surgery for Ischaemic Heart Disease

Any obstruction in the coronary arteries will impair the blood flow to the myocardium. Depending on how severe that impairment is, a number of consequences ranging from necrosis to mild ischaemia will occur. Ischaemic heart disease (IHD) accounts for about one-quarter of all deaths in the western world and a considerably larger burden of morbidity. Although there are many arterial lesions which may affect the coronary arteries, the commonest by far is atherosclerosis. The causes of this disease are not clear and so specific remedies are not available; all treatment is therefore palliative. Medical treatments have the broad aim of reducing the myocardial oxygen demands and surgical operations have the aim of increasing oxygen availability. Both medical and surgical approaches, however, have two ultimate aims in common: to reduce angina and to improve longevity.

Surgical objectives in IHD

There is still some residual controversy over whether medicine is more or less effective than surgery in achieving these aims. At the time of writing, however, it would appear that surgical operations which increase the blood supply offer better relief of symptoms and better longevity than medical treatments. None of the foregoing implies any lack of awareness of the importance of prevention of coronary atherosclerosis. Certain evidence exists that reduction of cigarette smoking, dietary modification and regular exercise are important preventive measures. However, most patients present with the established disease, the time of prevention being past. Vascular surgery in general is based on several principles:

1. Although atherosclerosis is a generalized arterial disease, it does have severe local obstructive features.
2. Rational surgery depends on the precise identification of these lesions by arteriography.
3. Restoration of the arterial flow to the tissues will only be of benefit if necrosis has not occurred.
4. Improvement of the blood supply by removal or bypassing of the lesions will cause an improvement which can be predicted by the amount of the increased flow.

Coronary arterial disease is thus a part of vascular disease in general. Nevertheless, the myocardium is a unique tissue both anatomically and physiologically and the consequences of IHD are therefore much more serious than ischaemia elsewhere. Surgical complications may occur:

1 During coronary arteriography.
2 During percutaneous transluminal angioplasty (PTCA).
3 Before cardiopulmonary bypass.
4 During cardiopulmonary bypass.
5 After cardiopulmonary bypass.

The major complication of IHD lies outside the surgeon's area of responsibility, i.e. necrosis of the left ventricle. There are many patients who have symptoms of IHD for many years, usually with several myocardial infarctions, who are referred for surgery only when there is widespread scarring and diminution of left ventricular function. No matter how well the surgery is performed, fibrous tissue will never return to contracting muscle and thus many patients cannot benefit from an operation. Such a complication can be prevented by earlier referral and this will only happen when an awareness of the benefits of surgery is appreciated. Surgeons play an important educational role in this matter.

In summary, the surgical treatment of IHD is palliative and aims to increase the blood supply to the myocardium. Surgery offers relief of angina and a reduction in the risk of infarction. The principles of surgery for IHD are identical to those of vascular surgery in general.

Surgical Complications of Coronary Arteriography

Precise identification of lesions in the coronary arteries can only be achieved by coronary arteriography. At the same time, the contractile state of the left ventricle and any scarring can be assessed by means of left ventriculography. Only when all evidence from both investigations is available can the risks of the disease, the exact nature of the surgical operation and the risks of that operation be assessed.

Coronary arteriography and left ventriculography are very commonly performed invasive investigations and are usually performed in the cardiac catheterization laboratory either by cardiologists or cardiac radiologists. The risks of the investigation are low – perhaps one untoward incident in every 5000 – provided that the investigator and the unit have sufficient experience and volume on a day-to-day basis.

Coronary arteriography and left ventriculography depend on the positioning of the catheter either in the coronary ostium or in the left ventricle. Access to the arterial system is needed either via the femoral artery (Judkin's technique) or via the brachial artery (Sones' technique). Usually, the brachial artery is visualized by a small incision over it. The femoral artery is usually cannulated percutaneously.

Surgical complications of coronary arteriography are:

1 Damage to the brachial or femoral artery.
2 Damage to the coronary arteries.
3 Haematoma over the access artery.

Damage to the brachial artery

This artery is usually healthy and once the catheter is passed dissection or tearing of the vessel is unusual. The commonest complication occurs when the catheter is removed and the arterial puncture repaired, usually with a pursestring suture. Occlusion of the artery may result and not be recognized at the time. After the investigation, the hand and forearm are obviously ischaemic being cold and lacking in both sensation and distal pulses.

Sometimes, there is a large element of spasm aggravating the physical obstruction to the brachial artery and it is permissible to spend a short time – perhaps up to one hour – waiting for spontaneous improvement to occur. If the signs of ischaemia are still present at that time, however, a formal exploration of the brachial artery should be performed. The artery should be controlled with tapes and opened at the site of the pursestring suture. Clot should be removed by use of the smallest balloon arterial catheter (Fogarty) and usually the incision repaired using a vein patch.

Damage to the femoral artery

The femoral artery is commonly affected by the atherosclerotic process. This usually begins as a posterior 'gutter' of atheroma and progresses to involve the whole artery. Percutaneous cannulation may dissect out the disease which then flaps down and obstructs the vessel. Thrombosis will eventually occur. Alternatively, the disease may prevent satisfactory haemostasis after the catheter is removed and a periarterial haematoma or even a false aneurysm may occur.

The investigator may fail to recognize that the cannula or catheter is not in the true lumen of the femoral vessel and forcibly push the catheter retrogradely, along the iliac vessels into the aorta, creating an iatrogenic dissection or even a rupture of these major vessels.

Ischaemia after femoral cannulation should lead to immediate exploration of the femoral artery. A wide exposure is needed to allow identification of the common femoral artery and its superficial and deep branches. The artery is controlled with tapes and opened at the site of puncture which is easily seen. Fresh thrombus and detached atheroma are usually found. Thrombus is removed by suction and by balloon-tipped catheter. A limited endarterectomy and vein patch are usually needed to restore femoral blood flow.

Dissection of the femoral or iliac arteries or the aorta will usually heal spontaneously once the catheter is removed. If there is persisting pain and guarding in the iliac fossa or in the abdomen, it is likely that rupture of the vessel has occurred, especially if there are signs of blood loss and oligaemia. In these circumstances, the aorta or iliac vessels should be exposed and the laceration directly repaired.

Damage to the coronary arteries (Fig. 8.1)

Coronary arteriography is performed by direct cannulation of the ostium of each coronary artery. To perform this from the brachial or femoral artery is an extremely skilled task given the normal variability of position and angle of the ostia. Trauma to the first part of the coronary artery may occur during this procedure but is rare and usually occurs when there is local disease. A flap of diseased arterial wall is lifted up into the lumen of the vessel and causes obstruction to flow. This process is called 'stripping' and is recognized radiologically by a partial or complete obstruction to flow in an artery previously shown to be normal at that point.

The action which needs to be taken depends on the response of the heart. Acute chest pain and electrocardiographic changes of ischaemia (acute ST segment depression) will lead to infarction if they persist for more than a few minutes. In this event, emergency coronary artery bypass grafting of the affected arteries should be performed. In the period of preparation, the heart will be helped by the support of the intra-aortic balloon inserted percutaneously in the catheter room.

Damage to the coronary arteries may occur unpredictably, even in the hands of the most experienced investigator. Coronary arteriography should not be performed unless there is an acute cardiac surgical unit within the same hospital prepared to deal rapidly with these rather rare emergencies.

Haematoma over the access artery

This complication affects mainly the femoral artery because of the percutaneous technique used to cannulate it and the fact that the artery is commonly diseased. When the catheters are removed from the artery, bleeding is controlled by digital pressure firmly applied for ten minutes as measured on the clock. Some degree of bruising around the puncture site is usual.

Occasionally, the pressure control may be inadequate or the arterial pressure unusually elevated. Also the diseased artery may tear slightly at the puncture site. A haematoma may then occur round the artery. Rarely, a false aneurysm follows.

A haematoma in the groin should be inspected on several occasions before deciding that it is not increasing in size. If an increase does occur, early exploration under local anaesthesia is

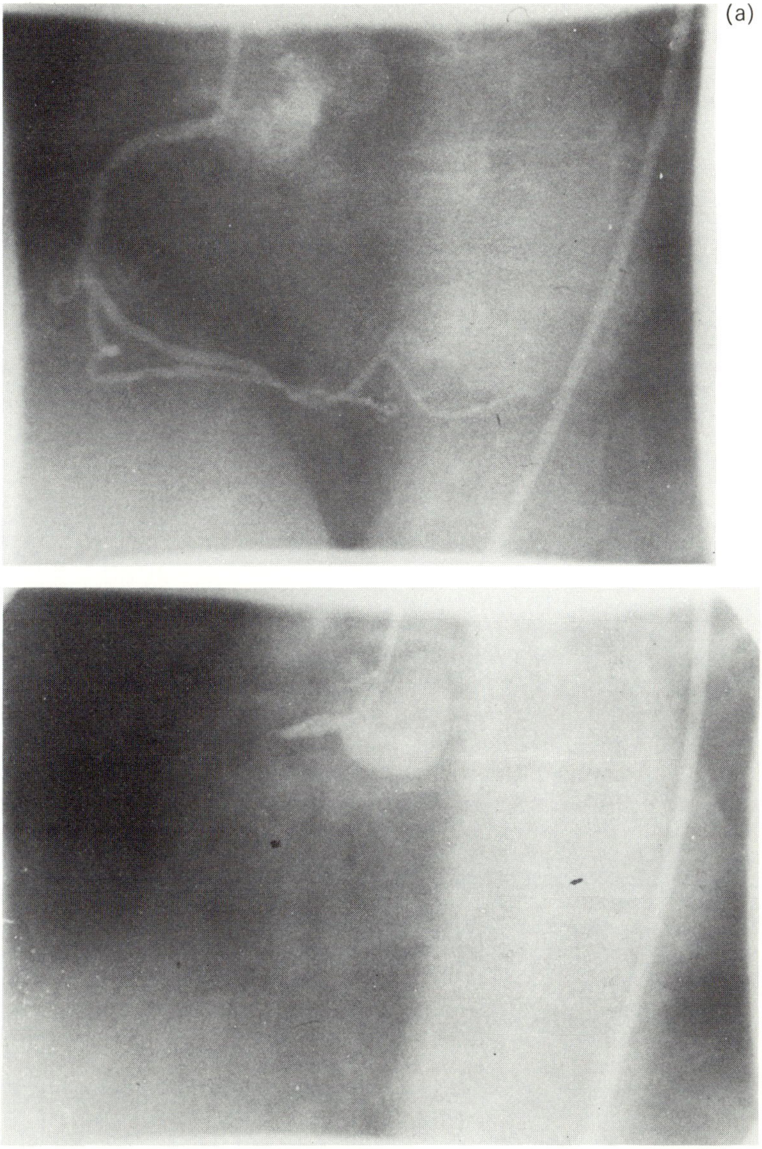

Figure 8.1
(a) Angiogram of the right coronary artery taken during a routine investigation. (b) Angiogram taken after same patient complained of severe chest pain during the procedure. Shows complete occlusion of the right coronary artery.

performed. Usually, a simple stitch will control the bleeding point on the artery. Exploration and evacuation of blood clot will reduce the morbidity of the large established haematoma which is not increasing in size.

The diagnosis of a false aneurysm in the femoral artery is not easy. Many haematomas have pulsation transmitted through them and it is not as easy as many textbooks claim to distinguish between intrinsic and transmitted pulsation in the groin. Any doubt should lead to exploration. If an aneurysm is found, it is dealt with by excision and repair of the femoral artery. If no aneurysm is found, the large haematoma can be evacuated and the period of morbidity reduced.

Summary

Coronary arteriography is a safe procedure in the hands of the experienced investigator. Damage to the access arteries or to the coronary arteries themselves leads to surgical complications. The treatment of these complications may have to be carried out urgently and it is important that cardiac surgical support is available.

The most common complication of coronary arteriography is a haematoma around the access artery. Surgical evacuation of large haematomas, although not absolutely indicated, will decrease the period of morbidity.

Persisting controversies

- Relative safety of Sones' or Judkin's techniques for coronary arteriography.
- Timing of surgery in large groin haematomas.

Surgical Complications During Percutaneous Transluminal Angioplasty of the Coronary Arteries (PTCA)

About 10% of all coronary artery stenoses are suitable for balloon dilatation carried out after coronary arteriography. In the most experienced hands, the stenoses can be abolished, pressure gradients reduced and blood flow down the coronary arteries greatly improved. Present evidence indicates that the dilated areas remain patent in the long term and give subjective and objective improvements in cardiac function.

The procedure involves the preliminary identification of the lesions by coronary arteriography. After this, the catheters are exchanged for a special balloon catheter which is inserted into the stenotic area and dilated. The surgical complications of this procedure are essentially those of coronary arteriography but with one major addition. Occasionally, the postdilatation arteriogram will show complete occlusion of the artery at the site of the original stenosis (Fig. 8.2). This is due to damage of the vessel wall leading to acute thrombosis. This event usually causes severe persisting chest pain, electrocardiographic changes and low cardiac output. If left, a myocardial infarction will result.

Before PTCA is performed, the cardiac surgical team should be informed and should be available. It is logistically wasteful for the team to be in a state of instant readiness with no other commitments. Instead, PTCA is performed during the course of the usual operating day. If a complication occurs, then it can be dealt with by rearranging the order of the operating list.

Figure 8.2
(a) Angiogram taken before PTCA showing severe stenosis of left anterior descending coronary artery. (b) Angiogram taken after attempt at PTCA in same patient. Total occlusion of the artery has occurred and this patient developed cardiac arrest. Successful surgical intervention was performed.

(a)

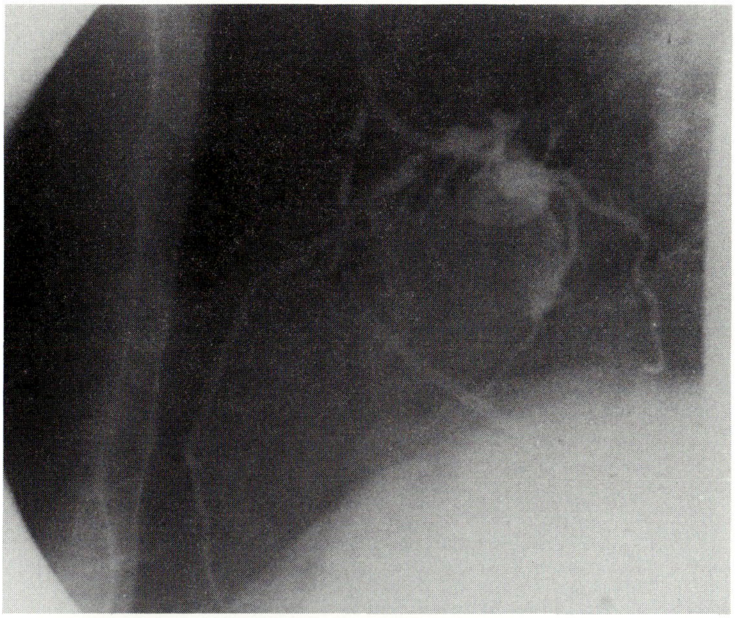

(b)

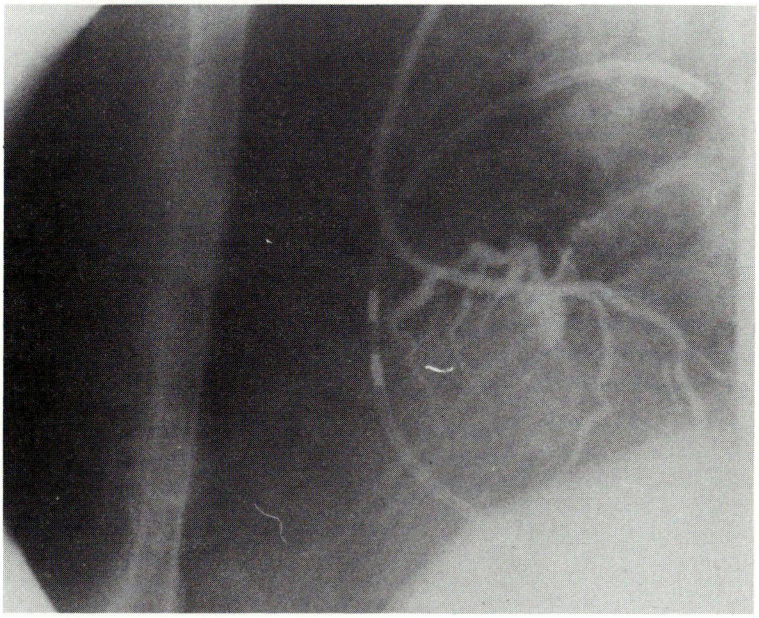

Emergency coronary artery bypass grafting is the remedy when this complication of PTCA occurs. Again, the support of the intra-aortic balloon pump will prevent or limit the amount of myocardial damage. During PTCA, the balloon pump is available in the catheter room, together with a range of percutaneous intra-aortic balloons.

Preoperative Complications of Coronary Arterial Surgery

The major preoperative complication of coronary arterial surgery is the occurrence of a myocardial infarction. This complication will greatly increase the risks of the operation and reduce the benefits even if the patient survives. In spite of the fact that the coronary arterial disease is severe and that the myocardium is in jeopardy, most infarcts at this stage are preventable by the proper medical management. Myocardial infarct should therefore be regarded as an iatrogenic complication when it occurs before surgical revascularization is accomplished.

Causes of preoperative myocardial infarction
(Table 8.1)

Changes in drug treatment. Patients presenting for coronary artery surgery have usually had full medical treatment for ischaemic heart disease, including vasodilators, β-blockers and calcium antagonists. Since both β-blockers and calcium antagonists have a myocardial depressant effect, it would seem desirable to stop them before surgery. However, there is evidence that the sudden cessation of these powerful drugs leads to an increased incidence of myocardial infarction and a worsening of the ischaemia. Indeed, there is good evidence to show that the continuation of β-blockers in particular leads to better preservation of myocardial function after surgery. The evidence for continuing calcium antagonists is less clear and some units discontinue these drugs before operation.

Disturbance in oxygen supply and demand. The complex factors determining oxygen supply and demand of the myocardium have already been described in the section on myocardial preservation (Chapter 5). Coronary arterial obstructions clearly introduce a further complication in this consideration, but the ischaemic heart may be so severely compromised that any increase in demand or reduction in supply will lead to critical ischaemia or frank myocardial necrosis. For instance, an elevated pulse rate and blood pressure will certainly worsen ischaemia and yet both may occur as a result of anaesthetic drugs or apprehension.

Table 8.1 Causes of preoperative myocardial infarction.

1 Changes in drug treatment
2 Disturbance in oxygen supply/demand ratio of the myocardium resulting from apprehension, anaesthetic drugs and surgical manipulation

Similarly, a short period of hypoxia during intubation may prove very damaging. As a further complication, the patient may be in no position to inform his doctors that chest pain is occurring. The ischaemia occurring after induction of anaesthesia will often lead to 'unexplained' cardiac arrest.

All these events conspire to make the period after arrival in the operating suite, and before being placed onto cardiopulmonary bypass, the most dangerous time during the whole of the hospital stay. Clearly, prevention of this complication is very important, together with its early recognition when it does occur.

Prevention of preoperative myocardial infarction

With the possible exception of calcium antagonists, all cardiac drugs should be continued up to the time of the operation. Indeed, a long-acting β-blocker may be chosen so as to give adequate levels at the time of surgery.

The patient should have his natural anxiety over the operation reduced by appropriate medication, beginning some 24 hours before surgery and finishing with a premedication which leaves him just rousable. The journey from his bed to the operating suite should be calm and unhurried and give rise to no apprehension on the patient's part.

On arrival in the operating suite, the radial artery is cannulated under local anaesthesia and an electrocardiogram attached before induction of anaesthesia. Many units also cannulate the internal jugular vein before anaesthesia. In this way, second-by-second knowledge of the arterial pressure, pulse rate and ECG is available together with access to central veins before anaesthesia is commenced. This knowledge permits accurate control of the various indices of myocardial oxygen availability and demand. Since the onset of ischaemia will increase the left atrial pressure, a minority of units also insert a balloon-tipped flotation catheter (Swann Ganz) before anaesthesia in those patients thought to be particularly at risk. All of these cannulations can be performed in a quiet room over a period of about ten minutes and although they might seem upsetting to the patient, they need not be so if suitable premedication is given and the tasks skilfully performed.

The period between induction of anaesthesia and the onset of cardiopulmonary bypass is dangerous even with knowledge and control of all the features of cardiac function. It is important that this time should be as short as possible. The patient should be anaesthetized in the operating theatre. During intubation, catheterization of the urinary bladder is performed simultaneously. Rapid preparation of the skin, draping of the chest and surgical exposure of the heart, followed by the cannulations for cardiopulmonary bypass, are then performed. In a critically ischaemic patient, the time from induction of anaesthesia to bypass can be reduced to about 16–20 minutes, but even in the low-risk patient should never exceed 30 minutes.

All of the above is in conflict with many of the established practices in the United Kingdom where there is a preference for unhurried preparation and anaesthesia, cannulations under the anaesthetic, and a leisurely surgical opening and mobilization of the chest, often by an inexperienced surgeon in training. Indeed, most patients will derive little direct benefit. However, even if one or two deaths are prevented every year, this will have the effect of reducing the mortality of this operation by some 50%.

Recognition of critical ischaemia in the prebypass period
The earliest reliable sign of ischaemia is a rising left atrial pressure and this can be detected by a balloon-tipped flotation catheter. This catheter is passed via a systemic vein, through the right atrium and ventricle into the pulmonary artery. It is then advanced until it impacts in a small pulmonary arteriole. The pressure then measured is called the 'wedge' pressure and is an indirect but fairly reliable indicator of left atrial pressure.

Clearly, a small number of patients are so ill that this measurement must be made, but in this small group, the early detection of critical ischaemia is crucial to avoid a myocardial infarction.

In most patients, an indirect left atrial pressure measurement probably carries more hazards than benefits. In this larger group, the first sign of increasing ischaemia will be ST segment depression in lead V_5 of the ECG and this is as reliable, if somewhat later, than the left atrial pressure elevation.

Later in the course of progressive ischaemia, there will be bradycardia and a falling cardiac output, usually followed by ventricular fibrillation, unless appropriate steps are taken.

Treatment of ischaemia in the prebypass period
The blood pressure and pulse rate should be adjusted so that the systolic arterial pressure is around 100 mgHg and the pulse rate between 80 and 100/min. A lower pressure will need elevating with a pure vasoconstrictor such as phenylephrine. Undue tachycardia will usually respond either to a deeper anaesthetic or small intravenous doses of a β-blocking drug such as propranolol (5 mg) or acebutolol (2.5 mg). Bradycardia will respond to calcium chloride (5 mmol i.v.) or isoprenaline (0.02 mg). Often, however, these measures will fail simply because of the severity of the coronary arterial disease. The only remedy then is to institute cardiopulmonary bypass as rapidly as possible.

There is a small group of patients who have unremitting angina in spite of all possible manoeuvres. Many surgeons insert an intra-aortic balloon before surgery so that the ischaemia is relieved and the prebypass period thereby made more safe. Other surgeons dislike this manoeuvre because of the dangers of the intra-aortic balloon.

Summary
The patient is at risk from critical ischaemia or myocardial infarction until the heart is supported by cardiopulmonary bypass. The period between induction of anaesthesia and bypass is particularly dangerous.

Preanaesthetic monitoring of the cardiovascular system, expeditious surgery, and control of the arterial pressure and the pulse rate are essential to avoid provoking ischaemia.

Persisting controversies
- Preanaesthetic cannulation of the radial artery and insertion of the central venous pressure line.
- Abandoning the anaesthetic room.
- The indications for the insertion of a balloon-tipped flotation catheter before anaesthesia.

Complications Occurring During Cardiopulmonary Bypass

Once the heart is supported by total cardiopulmonary bypass, there is no danger of critical ischaemia occurring, provided the perfusion pressure stays above (say) 40 mmHg. The method of myocardial protection employed is at the discretion of the surgeon, the two most widely practised techniques being hypothermic hyperkalaemic cardioplegia, or intermittent fibrillation and cross-clamping of the aorta.

The objective is to bypass all significant stenoses of major coronary vessels. The definition of 'significant' is a 50% or greater stenosis of a vessel, but this is not a precise measurement. The most common conduit used to bypass the lesions is a saphenous vein harvested from the leg and reversed. Veins from the arms, and the internal mammary artery which may be mobilized from the retrosternal tissues, can also be used. Synthetic conduits are not widely used and are of unproven value at the time of writing. With all conduits, apart from the internal mammary artery, the proximal end is anastomosed to the ascending aorta and the distal end to the coronary artery distally to each lesion. Precise identification of each vessel and the site of its lesion are essential before the operation and each vessel so affected should be bypassed.

Clearly, with such small vessels (1–3 mm) the techniques of anastomosing the vein to the artery or aorta have to be precise; this process is aided by a still heart, a bloodless field and optical magnification. Nearly all surgeons use polypropylene for anastomosis, but there are many variations of technique – the one shown (Fig. 8.3) is one of several available. Most surgeons perform all distal (i.e. vein-to-coronary artery) anastomoses first and then, with the heart perfused and beating but still on bypass,

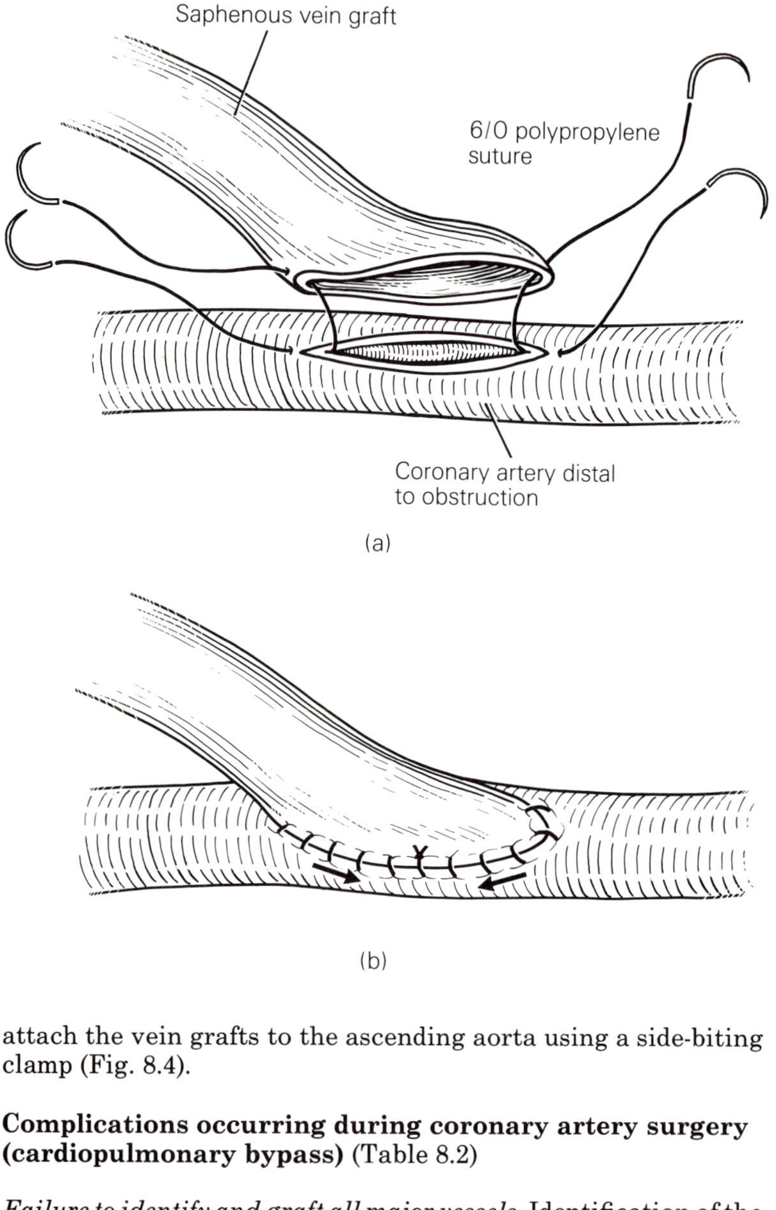

Figure 8.3
One method of performing the vein-to-artery anastomosis during coronary artery surgery.

attach the vein grafts to the ascending aorta using a side-biting clamp (Fig. 8.4).

Complications occurring during coronary artery surgery (cardiopulmonary bypass) (Table 8.2)

Failure to identify and graft all major vessels. Identification of the coronary arteries may be made difficult by epicardial fat or by muscle. Nevertheless, with constant reference to the cine angiogram, which should be available in or near to the operating theatre, every major vessel can and must be identified. Great patience may be required to achieve this objective.

Faulty opening of the coronary artery (Fig. 8.5). The artery should be opened longitudinally by a clean incision distal to the

Figure 8.4
(a) Ascending aorta with a side-biting clamp applied and holes made for upper ends of vein graft to be attached. (b) Vein graft being attached to ascending aorta. (c) Vein grafts attached to ascending aorta (operation completed).

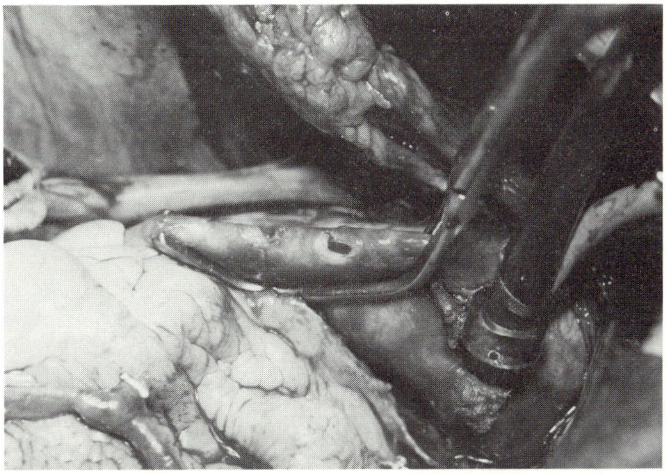

(a)

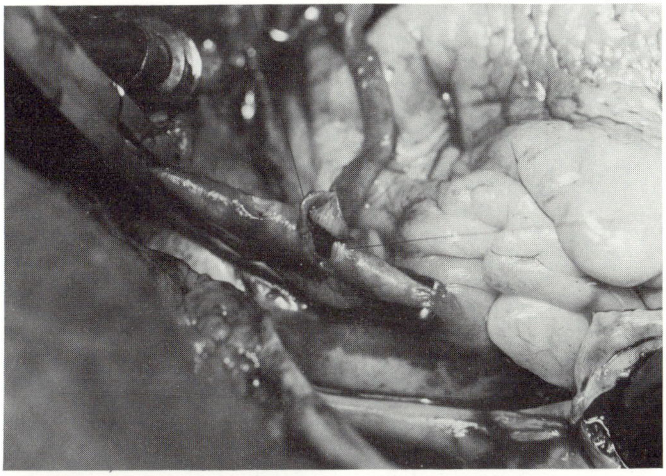

(b)

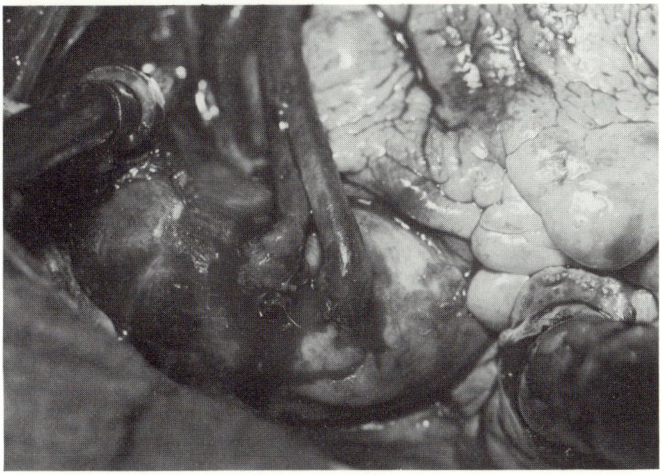

(c)

Table 8.2
Complications occurring during coronary artery surgery (cardiopulmonary bypass).

1 Failure to identify and graft all affected vessels
2 Faulty opening of the coronary artery
3 Failure to ensure adequate 'run-off'
4 Occlusion of the native coronary artery by the venoarterial anastomosis
5 Twisting or kinking of the vein
6 Too short a vein
7 Difficulties with the aortovenous anastomosis

obstruction. The length of the incision need not be greater than three times the diameter of the artery and very often less than this. After opening, the artery should be probed with graduated probes so that the distal arterial tree is seen to be free of disease. Should the artery be opened at the site of disease, the atheroma needs to be removed by endarterectomy which carries some hazards. If the probe fails to pass distally, there is peripheral disease and a further vein graft needs to be placed distally.

Failure to ensure an adequate 'run-off'. 'Run-off' means that the flow which is delivered by an arterial graft is actually getting to the capillaries. A good run-off provides a satisfactory solution to ischaemia. A poor run-off leads to early occlusion of the graft because of low flow. The position of the insertion of the graft on the coronary artery will clearly influence the run-off, but sometimes there may be distal disease of a diffuse nature which impairs the run-off. There may be little the surgeon can do about this apart from endarterectomy.

Occlusion of the native coronary artery by the venoarterial anastomosis (Fig. 8.6). This is clearly a technical problem and can be avoided by careful technique and probing of the anastomosis immediately before completion. This complication usually causes a fatal myocardial infarction.

Twisting or kinking of the vein will lead to an obstruction of the flow and early occlusion of the graft. Great attention is needed to prevent this complication and marking of the vein along its length with a dye will help. Kinking of the vein is due to an excessive length being used and is avoidable by careful measurement on the beating heart before bypass.

Too short a vein is also avoided by careful measurements on the beating heart. If a vein is too short when attached, a segment of extra vein is inserted by venovenous anastomosis.

Summary During bypass, complications are related to the technical aspects of the operation. Meticulous and prolonged attention to the

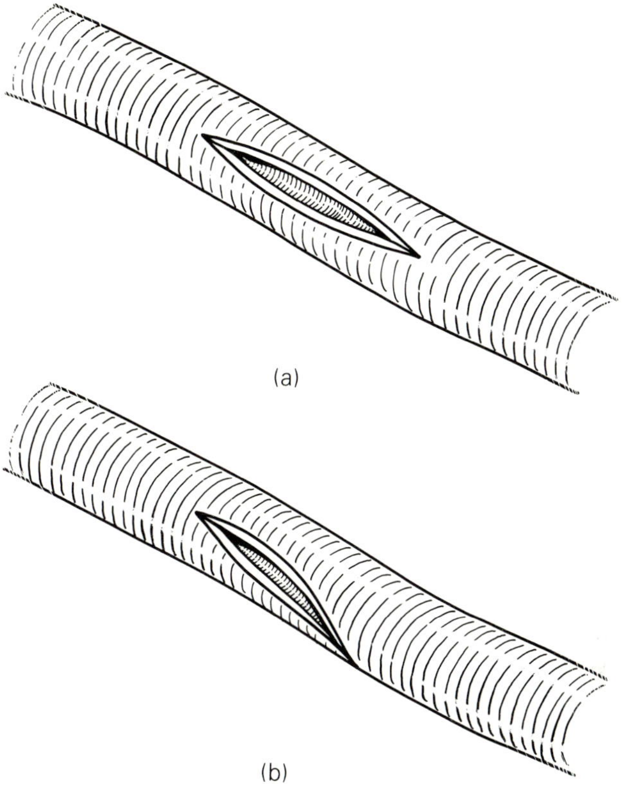

Figure 8.5
(a) Ideal way to open a coronary artery for grafting. (b) An incision which will create technical difficulties and lead to early obstruction of the graft.

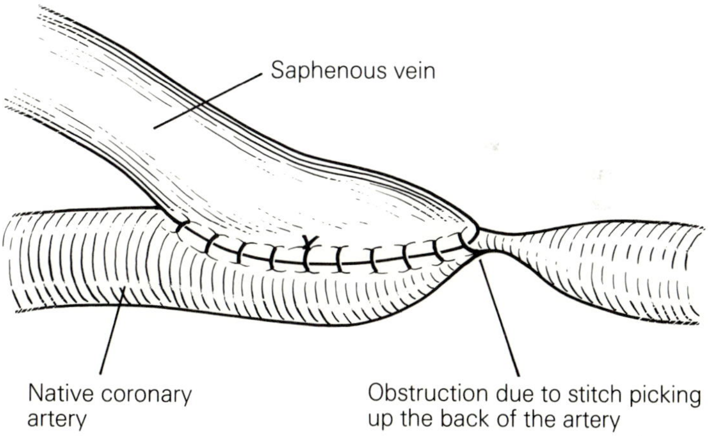

Figure 8.6
A carelessly placed deep stitch at the apex of the lower anastomosis will narrow the native vessel and predispose to early obstruction.

performance of distal and proximal anastomoses, the positioning of vein grafts and, above all, the accurate identification (and bypass graft) of all major diseased arteries is essential.

Persisting controversies

- The best way of performing the proximal and distal anastomoses.

- The place of optical magnification.
- Endarterectomy of diseased major vessels as opposed to multiple distal grafts.

Complications occurring after cardiopulmonary bypass for coronary artery bypass grafting (CABG)

Usually the heart resumes action very well when the bypass ends after coronary grafting. The ischaemia is abolished and the muscle responds immediately to the increased inflow of blood. The period between the end of bypass and the final closure of the chest is the most trouble-free of the whole operation but complications may occasionally happen (Table 8.3).

Cardiac failure after CABG

When the bypass finishes, the cardiac action may be obviously sluggish and there may be evidence of a poor cardiac output. If this is associated with a raised pulmonary artery pressure, as judged by the finger, cardiac failure is present.

Causes of cardiac failure after CABG (Table 8.4)

Inadequate revascularization. If a major part of the myocardium is ischaemic at the end of a CABG operation, there will be an inadequate cardiac action. Clearly, the operation should be performed with the angiogram in mind and every major vessel which has a significant stenosis must be grafted. Repeated reference to the angiogram may be necessary during the operation and the vessels themselves may be difficult to find if they lie under muscle or fat. No matter how difficult a vessel is to find, a prolonged search must be made and continued until successful identification is achieved. There are several aids to identifying 'deep' arteries. First, the myocardium over a deep artery often has an external groove lying over the course of the artery. Second, there may be a white or more pale area along the line of the artery. Dissection of these areas will not only reveal the vessel on many occasions, but when found the vessel is usually large and with healthy walls.

Inadequate revascularization may occur because the grafts fail

Table 8.3 Complications occurring after cardiopulmonary bypass for CABG.

1	Cardiac failure
2	Bleeding from the suture lines
3	Unsatisfactory positioning of the grafts

Table 8.4 Causes of cardiac failure after CABG.

1	Inadequate revascularization
2	Intraoperative myocardial damage
3	Metabolic causes
4	Undiagnosed cardiac lesions

to deliver a satisfactory volume of blood. The major reason for this is technical and may be avoided by probing all grafts before closure to ensure patency. The grafts may be too short or too long and the tension or kinking caused may impair blood flow along them. Attention to the proper length of the graft is important, but the decisions are not easy to make. Ideally, the lengths of the grafts should be measured on the beating working heart before bypass, but often this is not possible. Even if the graft length is adjusted before the proximal end is anastomosed to the aorta, great care is needed especially with grafts supplying the back of the heart.

Intraoperative myocardial damage. Myocardial damage inflicted during CABG is iatrogenic and avoidable in most cases. There is, however, no agreement as to the best method of myocardial protection. Most surgeons, especially those in training, prefer the quiet, bloodless conditions given by cardioplegia. There are many skilled and experienced surgeons, however, who both subjectively and objectively achieve the same high level of protection by using intermittent induced ventricular fibrillation and if necessary ischaemic arrest. Either method, if properly performed, is therefore likely to be adequate. If any damage does occur, it is likely to be reversible after a few minutes total cardiopulmonary bypass and rest.

Metabolic causes. Some patients have a failing heart because of acidosis, but this is not a feature specific to coronary bypass operations. However, treatment with β-blockers is specific and most patients are taking these drugs before operation. That depression of cardiac action rarely occurs is perhaps surprising. However, some β-blockers (such as propranolol) do have an indirect cardiac depressing action. These drugs can inhibit the peripheral utilization of potassium ions and the serum potassium level rises during bypass to reach levels (6.5 mmol/l or more) which are extremely depressing to the myocardium. Consequently, if the heart fails after a CABG operation, the concentration of serum potassium must be checked. If higher than 5.0 mmol/l, it should be lowered by the infusion of insulin and glucose (40 ml 50% dextrose with 20 units of soluble insulin).

Temporary myocardial failure may occur if air embolism to the coronary arteries occurs. This complication may be avoided by only allowing the flow along grafts to begin when the air in them has been removed by a fine needle.

Treatment of cardiac failure after CABG

Rather than driving the heart with inotropic drugs, bypass should be restarted when the problem is identified. This allows the heart to be reperfused in a beating non-working state and allows repayment of any oxygen debt.

While bypass is in progress, the acid–base state and concentration of serum potassium is measured and corrected if necessary. The grafts are needled to release any air they may contain. Inspection of the grafts may reveal unsatisfactory lengths and these should be corrected, if necessary, by shortening or lengthening the grafts. If the quality of an anastomosis is suspect, the vein is opened on one of its side branches and carefully probed. If occlusion has occurred, the anastomosis must be taken down and repeated. Failure of graft to work because of an inadequate run-off caused by peripheral coronary disease may be detected if the flow along a graft is poor, and an electromagnetic flow meter is useful at detecting this. The solution to peripheral disease is difficult, however, since surgery may be impossible. Nevertheless, peripheral disease is an uncommon cause of poor flow in a graft; poor anastomoses are much more common and the solution to this problem lies within the surgeon's ability.

If the heart still functions badly when all causes have been excluded and bypass finished, cardiac support is needed. Inotropic drugs and calcium may improve the heart and the improvement sustained. However, the outlook for such a patient is unsatisfactory because the cause of such a state is usually severe myocardial damage. The use of vasodilators and the intra-aortic balloon pump may help. The ideal answer is to avoid the situation in the first place. This can be done by careful selection of patients, careful surgery and meticulous myocardial protection.

Bleeding from suture lines

This complication may be apparent during the operation, or it may only declare itself later when the patient is in the recovery ward. Persistent bleeding from the top or bottom anastomosis of a vein graft arises as a result of technical inadequacy, often in the face of diseased vessels. The remedy is to identify the bleeding point and suture it. Three problems arise: first, the stitch has to be inserted blindly and, if at the 'toe' or 'heel' of the distal anastomosis, may occlude the native vessel; second, the vessels are under pressure and may tear as the extra stitch is put in and tied; finally, access to the bleeding point may distort the heart so much that its action fails.

Inspection of all anastomoses should be meticulously performed before the cannulas of the cardiopulmonary bypass are removed. If a bleeding point is found, the bypass may be temporarily restarted and the extra stitch put in under the most favourable circumstances. After decannulation, bleeding is more troublesome. Distal anastomosis bleeding should be treated by inserting an extra stitch after temporary clamping of the vein graft. Bleeding from the aortic end of a graft also needs suturing, but the aortic pressure must be reduced. This can be most safely achieved by temporarily cross-clamping the inferior vena cava with the pericardium. This manoeuvre safely reduces the aortic pressure by half and allows sutures to be placed without the aortic wall tearing.

Bleeding may occur from side branches of the vein graft which have not been controlled. Once this problem is identified, a simple pursestring suture will easily give control.

Unsatisfactory positioning of the grafts

This is a complication which may not interfere with cardiac action and yet tends to produce early occlusion of the grafts in the weeks or months after surgery. The cause lies in too long a graft being placed on the heart. As the chest is closed, the vein kinks and ultimately thrombosis will occur.

If a graft is extremely long, it should be shortened and reattached to the ascending aorta. If the graft is less long, the excess length may be accommodated by stitching the graft onto the epicardium in a sinuous manner so that no kinks occur.

Summary

After completion of cardiopulmonary bypass during a coronary bypass operation, cardiac failure, bleeding or unsatisfactory positioning of the vein grafts may be apparent.

Cardiac failure has several possible causes, but inadequate revascularization, myocardial damage and metabolic disturbances may be present. While the cause of the problem is identified, the heart should be supported by resuming cardiopulmonary bypass. If the cause is identified and reversed, the prognosis is good. However, inotropic support and possibly intra-aortic balloon pumping, although effective in the short term, often lead to unsatisfactory results in the absence of an identified remediable problem.

Bleeding is always surgical and needs extra sutures to be inserted to stop it. Care must be taken not to occlude the native coronary artery.

Unsatisfactory positioning of the vein grafts may not cause complications during the operation but may only be identified and remedied at that time.

Persisting controversies

- The ideal method of myocardial protection during CABG operations.
- The necessity for left ventricular decompression (LV venting) during CABG operations.

Postoperative Complications of CABG (Table 8.5)

Low output syndrome

This syndrome is discussed fully on page 78 and its management is along the lines already described. However, a general statement specific to ischaemic heart surgery may be made here. Persistent low output after correction of hypovolaemia is most commonly due to myocardial infarction or cardiac tamponade. Since there is no completely sensitive and specific way to distinguish between these two conditions after cardiac surgery,

Table 8.5
Postoperative complications of CABG.

1 Low output syndrome
2 Bleeding
3 Arrhythmias
4 Myocardial infarction

there should be no hesitation in reopening the chest if the low output persists or worsens.

Bleeding
This is nearly always 'surgical' and comes from an anastomotic suture line or side branch of the vein graft. Early exploration is indicated.

Arrhythmias
A tachycardia of up to 110/min in sinus rhythm is common after a coronary operation, probably because of lessening of β-blockade. Beyond this level, hypoxia, hypovolaemia, tamponade and pain must be excluded. Many surgeons commence a low dose of blocker after operation in an effort to reduce and minimize tachycardia. Other more disturbing arrhythmias are discussed in Chapter 12.

Myocardial infarction
If this complication occurs after coronary artery surgery, it may be difficult to document and only serial estimations of the M.B. isoenzyme of creatinine phosphokinase are reliable and sufficiently sensitive. If diagnosed, the patient should be treated as any medical patient on the coronary care unit.

Complications of Harvesting the Vein Graft

As already stated, most coronary operations use a vein as the grafting tissue and usually that vein is taken from the patient's legs or perhaps arms during the same operation. The short- and long-term success of the operation depends on the ability of the vein to act as a conduit at aortic pressure without occluding (Table 8.6). It is surprising, therefore, that the vein is usually harvested by the least experienced member of the surgical team, operating with the least help under difficult circumstances.

The high pressure to which vein grafts are subjected when in place is clearly unavoidable. Nevertheless, the manner in which the vein is dissected and prepared may be a source of avoidable trauma. This may arise in several ways:

1 Handling with metallic instruments.
2 Excessive traction during dissection.
3 Excessively high inflation pressures during preparation (150 + mmHg).

Table 8.6
Causes of vein graft occlusion.

1 Poor flow
2 Thrombosis due to both trauma and as a response to high blood pressure
3 Subintimal and medial thickening, and fibrosis due to high pressure and possibly operative trauma
4 Atherosclerotic changes in the wall of the vein, the causes of which are not known but which are accelerated in the presence of blood lipid abnormalities

All of these factors dispose to intimal damage and this progresses in many cases to fibrin deposition and ultimate thrombosis. The skill and experience of the surgeon harvesting the vein will determine how much trauma is inflicted, and in many centres the most experienced surgeon removes the vein while the assistant opens the patient's chest.

Most surgeons begin by mobilizing the long saphenous vein at the ankle (Fig. 8.7a). The vein is divided and its distal end ligated. The proximal vein is then cannulated and gently distended with saline or heparinized blood (Fig. 8.7b). The dissection of the vein proceeds proximally, side branches being identified and controlled with ligatures or metal clips.

In the shin, the saphenous nerve runs alongside the vein. Care should be taken to identify and preserve this nerve as damage to it causes paraesthesia and pain which persist for months after surgery. Preservation of the nerve is often made difficult by its being twisted around the saphenous vein (Fig. 8.8).

During the dissection, care must be taken to incise the skin directly over the vein. If skin flaps are created by undermining the skin, necrosis of the wound edges will occur.

As the dissection proceeds proximally, the saphenous vein at first becomes more superficial, with many tributaries around the knee, and then becomes quite deeply placed in the thigh. When the vein is removed, it should be gently flushed and placed in heparinized blood until required. Many surgeons mark the vein with dye to avoid it becoming twisted during positioning on the heart. Closure of the leg wound should be performed in two layers and often it will be necessary to drain the thigh wound with one or two suction drains. At the conclusion of the operation, the leg is elevated and a crêpe bandage firmly applied.

Before the vein is used, it should be gently inflated and any residual leaks repaired using a fine suture; these are placed in such a way that the main lumen of the vein is not in any way reduced. Varicosities occurring along the vein should be excluded from the grafts or, if this is impossible, a sleeve of extra vein should be passed over the graft so as to support the varicosity (Fig. 8.9).

Summary

The harvesting and preparation of the vein for CABG is an

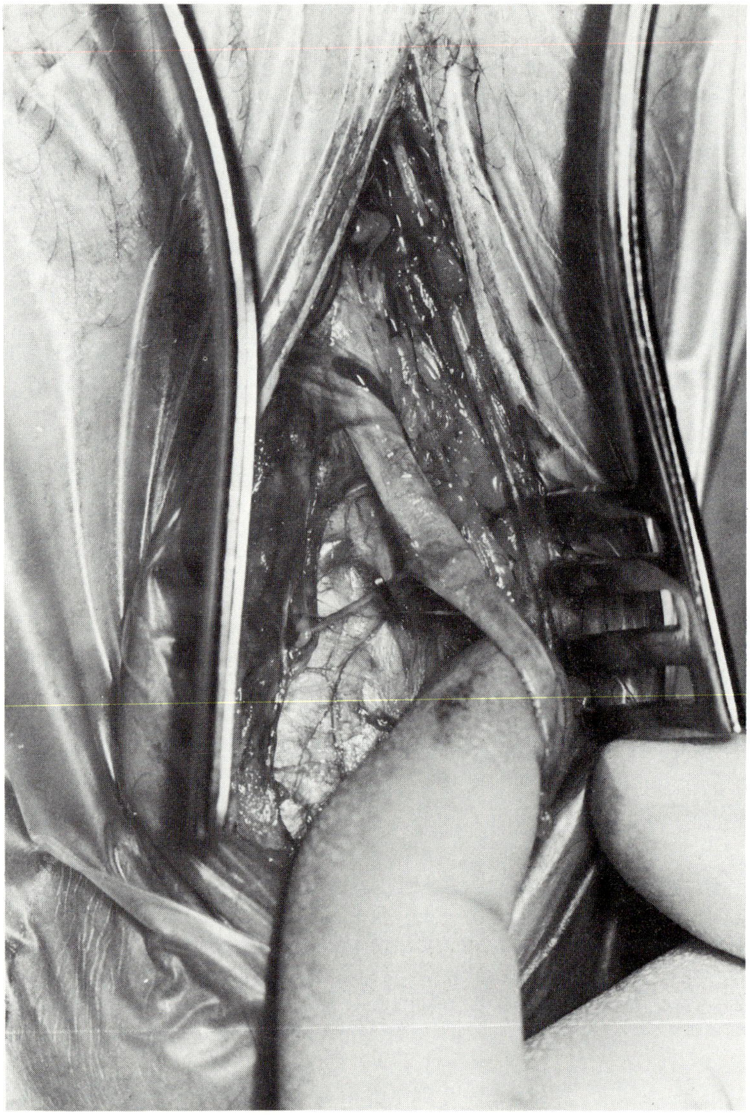

(a)

Figure 8.7
(a) Beginning of harvest of saphenous vein. Note handling of vein gently with finger – no forceps used. (b) (opposite) Vein has been mobilized and about to be gently distended with saline.

important part of the operation because trauma may be inflicted which will lead to occlusion of the graft later. Careful dissection and the avoidance of excessive distension pressures will minimize intimal damage. From the vein available, grafts should be prepared only from the most healthy parts.

Persisting controversies

- The ideal solution for flushing and distending vein grafts – blood or saline.
- The best way to avoid excessive distension pressures.

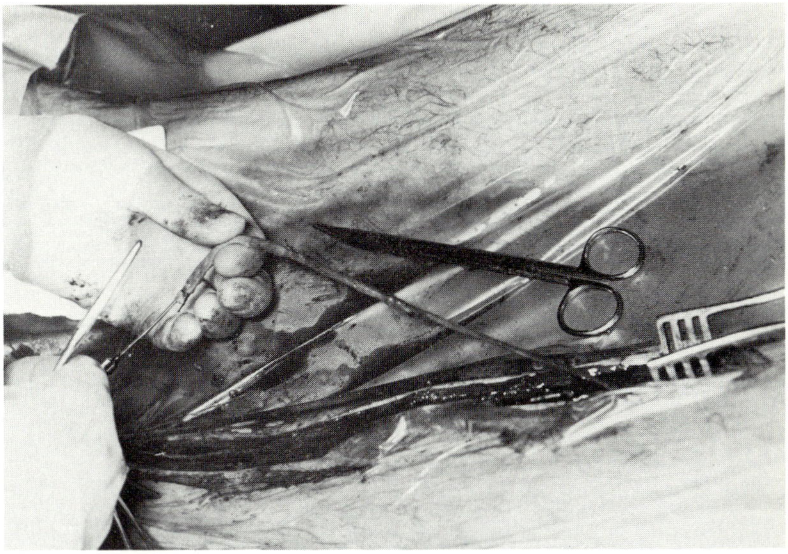

Figure 8.7 (b)

Late Postoperative Complications of Coronary Bypass Operations

About one-sixth of all vein grafts will occlude within the first year of operation. Thereafter, the grafts tend to remain open, but there will be a small percentage of occlusions occurring all the time. Occlusion of vein grafts is due to the following causes (see also Table 8.6):

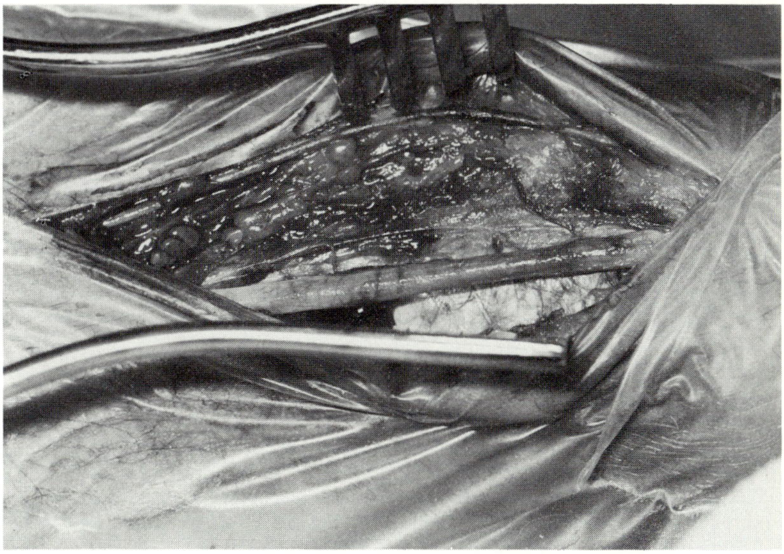

Figure 8.8 Saphenous vein closely accompanied by saphenous nerve which should be identified and preserved.

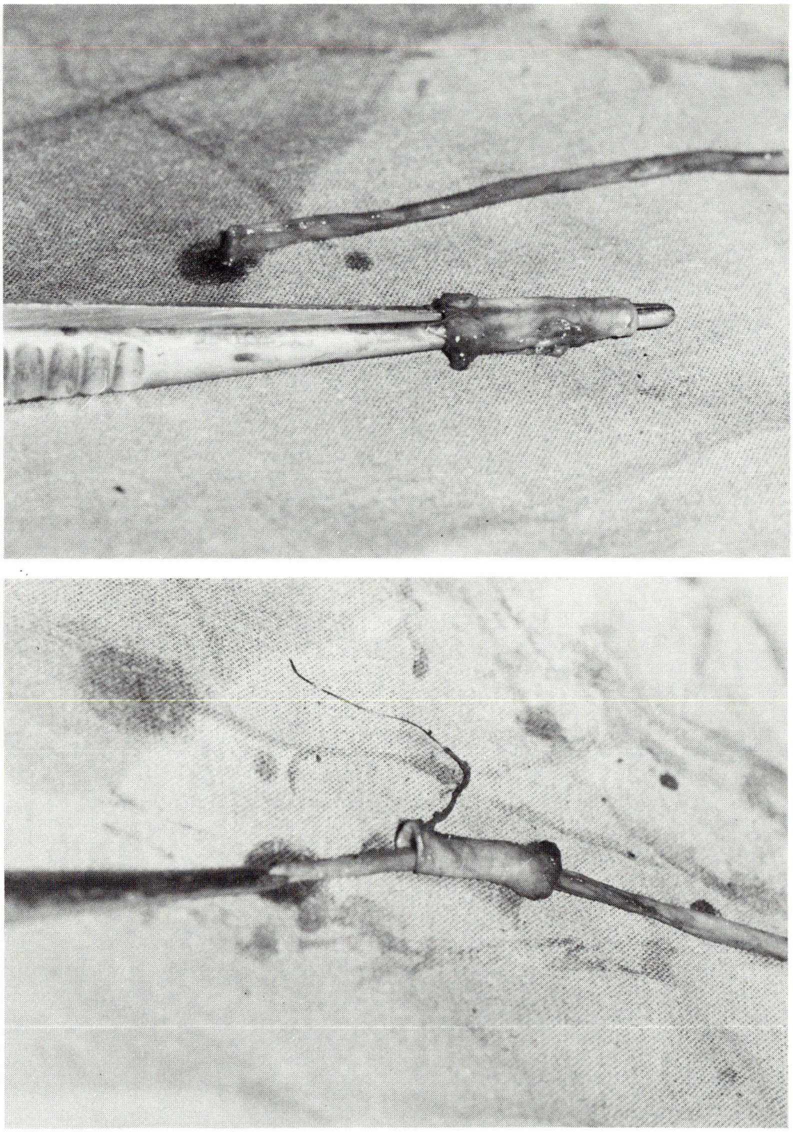

Figure 8.9
(a) Larger but normal vein taken to protect a varicosity in the graft. (b) Segment is teased over varicosity and secured by a few superficial stitches.

1 Poor run-off due to either peripheral disease in the grafted artery or obstruction at the anastomosis.
2 Thrombosis in the graft due to the changes in the wall already described or due to kinking of the graft.

The run-off of the graft can be improved at the time of operation by using a meticulous technique and by inserting the graft onto large, healthy, distal arteries. Thrombosis in the graft due to wall changes is only partly under the surgeon's control. Careful preparation and positioning of the vein are effective, but the degree of wall change will also depend on non-surgical factors. There is good evidence that antiplatelet drugs help to maintain graft patency. Dipyridamole (100 mg three times daily) and acetylsalicylic acid (300 mg once daily) have been shown to be very effective in combination, *if* started before surgery and continued indefinitely afterwards.

Early chest pain after CABG

This symptom may arise from the following causes:

1 Myocardial ischaemia due to occlusion of grafts.
2 Wound and sternal pain.
3 Pleural pain.
4 Postcardiotomy pain.

To distinguish between these causes may be very difficult. A careful history may show that the pain has anginal characteristics, in particular being rapidly relieved by sublingual trinitrates. Wound and sternal pain are often postural and the most severe pain is felt when the patient turns over in bed at night. Pleural pain sometimes occurs after the pleura has been opened during operation and blood has found its way into the pleural cavity. Distinguishing pleuritic pain from wound pain is often impossible from the history. Postcardiotomy pain is usually associated with general malaise.

Examination is only a little more helpful. Tenderness over the wound and provoking the symptoms by 'springing' the chest wall suggest wound problems. A pleural rub may be present after a small haemothorax.

Most patients give a rather vague history of chest pain and examination is unrewarding. Since the original operation was for relief of chest pain, its persistence or occurrence is a matter of anxiety to the patient and may distort the judgement of his doctor. Ultimately, the most difficult or persistent cases will have to undergo further cardiac investigations. Exercise ECG and thallium screening tests may suggest areas of ischaemic myocardium and subsequently arteriography or 'graftgrams' should be performed. Only in this way can the patency of the grafts be established and an end put to speculation.

If the pain is ischaemic, and has been shown to be due to blocked grafts, medical and surgical options of treatment should be reviewed.

Late chest pain after CABG

Chest pain recurring more than one year after a coronary artery bypass operation may be due to the following causes:

1 Closure of the grafts.
2 Progression of the native disease.

Wound and other chest wall problems rarely recur at a period greater than one year after surgery. Closure of the grafts due to degenerative changes in the vein wall still occurs although at a much lower rate than in the first year. The native disease which of course has only been bypassed at the original operation, has usually progressed.

There is no clinical way of identifying the cause of late chest pain. If exercise ECG and/or thallium scans suggest ischaemia of the myocardium, coronary arteriography and 'graftgrams' are needed. Depending on the information gained, a rationally based management can be started.

Progression of the native disease is inevitable and since the causes of atherosclerosis in general are unknown, it is impossible to give any specific treatments or preventive measures. However, some modifications of the patient's way of living after a CABG operation may have an influence on the rate of progression of the disease. Patients are strongly advised not to smoke tobacco and to remain slim. A gentle exercise programme is probably also of benefit. Those patients with a demonstrable lipid abnormality of the blood should have it treated appropriately. With the exception of this latter action, it must be re-emphasized that all the other strategies listed are of marginal importance at best in slowing the disease process.

Summary

Chest pain may occur early or late after CABG. Early chest pain occurring in the first year may be due to several causes apart from myocardial ischaemia and chest wall pain may be very difficult to distinguish from recurrent angina. After the first year, recurrent chest pain is nearly always due to myocardial ischaemia. Full invasive investigation is the only way to tell if there has been occlusion of vein grafts or progression of the disease. Once the cause of chest pain is established, treatment can be given on the merits of the individual. Measures designed to slow down the atherosclerotic process are of doubtful benefit.

Persisting controversies

- The usefulness of exercise ECG screening in the non-invasive investigation of postCABG chest pain.
- The duration of antiplatelet treatment after operation.
- The timing of coronary arteriography in recurrent chest pain postCABG.

Further reading

Braunwald, E. (1977) Coronary artery surgery at the crossroads (Editorial). *N. Engl. J. Med.*, *297*, 661.

DeLaria, G.A., Hunter, J.A., Goldin, M.D., Serry, C., Javid, H. & Najafi, H. (1981) Leg wound complications associated with coronary revascularization. *J. Thorac. Cardiovasc. Surg.*, *81*, 403.

Favoloro, R.E. (1969) Saphenous vein graft in the surgical treatment of coronary artery disease; operative technique. *J. Thorac. Cardiovasc. Surg.*, *56*, 253.

Favoloro, R.E. (1970) *Surgical Treatment of Coronary Arteriosclerosis*. Baltimore: Williams and Wilkins.
Grondin, C.M., Castonguay, Y.R., Lesperance, J., Borassa, M.J., Campeau, L. & Grondin, P. (1972) Attrition rate of aorta-to-coronary artery saphenous vein grafts after one year. *Ann. Thorac. Surg.*, *14*, 223.
Ullyot, D.J. (1980) Current controversies in the conduct of the coronary bypass operation. *Ann. Thorac. Surg.*, *30*, 192.
Vlodover, Z. & Edwards, J.E. (1971) Pathologic changes in aortic coronary arterial saphenous vein grafts. *Circulation*, *44*, 719.

9 Complications of Surgery for Congenital Heart Disease

Approximately six of every thousand live births will have some form of congenital heart disease. Some of these lesions are very severe and kill the child in a matter of hours or days. Others are less severe and permit good function and survival for many years. Thus, surgical operations may be indicated at any age on strictly medical criteria. However, the disruption of a child's normal development and education which is entailed in lengthy investigations and possible surgery dictates that early treatment is best for the individual child. In addition, the burdens of congenital heart disease often interrupt normal growth and place strain on other organ systems. For these reasons, there is an increasing trend towards the investigation and treatment of congenital heart disease at an early age. As the skills and knowledge of those looking after these children have increased, so the age at which intervention is considered to be safe has fallen.

There is also a tendency, if possible, towards corrective surgery instead of palliative surgery which usually involves several operations. Ideally, therefore, children with heart disease should be operated on before going to school and a 'corrective' operation should be performed. The more severe lesions will be operated on in the first two years of life in order to promote normal development thereafter.

This ideal has led to a number of surgical units specializing in the cardiac surgery of children in the first two years of life. Children of this age are often very sick and require the combined and constant attention of paediatricians, cardiologists, anaesthetists and surgeons with appropriately trained and experienced nursing staff. Paediatric cardiac surgery has therefore tended to become, for the best of reasons, a specialty in its own right. It is beyond the scope of this book to deal with this subject in the detail it deserves. Instead, this chapter will outline the complications of the surgery of congenital heart disease falling outside the specialized group. A further justification of this approach is that over 70% of all congenital heart disease will be treated after the first two years of life.

The surgery of most congenital heart lesions will continue to be performed in units where the broad range of cardiothoracic surgery occurs. Most of the lesions are essentially simple and their correction straightforward. Nevertheless, children are not small adults and there must be close co-operation with paediatricians over all aspects of the care of these children. Thus, the organizational aspects of this sort of cardiac surgery are very important and need to be established long before the patient has an operation.

Complications of Closed Cardiac Operations for Congenital Heart Disease

Persistent ductus arteriosus (PDA) (Fig. 9.1)
The ductus usually closes within a few days of birth. Its persistence leads to a flow of blood from the aorta to the pulmonary artery because of pressure difference. Depending on the size of the ductus, there will be an excessive blood flow through the lungs and strain on the left ventricle which has to maintain a higher than normal output. Ultimately, left heart failure and pulmonary vascular damage will occur. Another danger is that the ductus may be the seat of endocarditis. PDA accounts for approximately 13% of congential heart disease.

Surgical closure of the ductus is safe and can therefore be recommended early in life. The operation is performed as a 'closed' procedure through the left chest. After controlling the aorta with tapes, the ductus is doubly ligated or occasionally

Figure 9.1
Anatomy of the persistent ductus arteriosus.

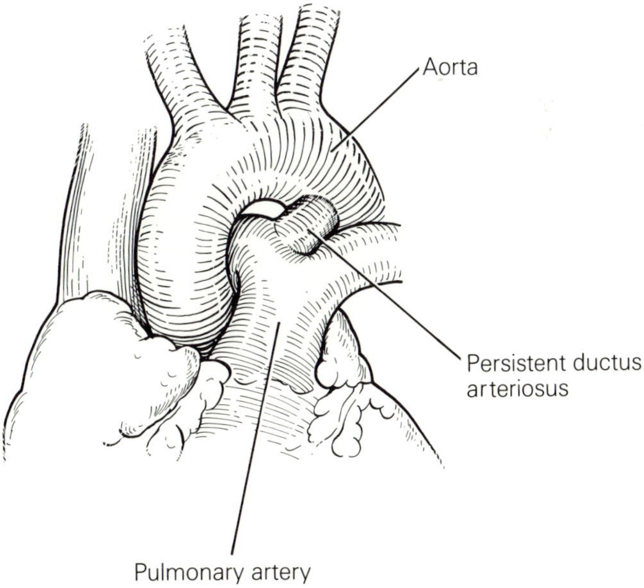

divided. The complications of closure of PDA, as discussed below, are listed in Table 9.1.

Failure to close the PDA

This is usually a failure of the ligation technique, although it can happen when a structure other than the PDA, such as an abnormally sited right subclavian artery or a secondary aortic arch, is divided instead of the PDA. Failure to obliterate the PDA is diagnosed when the flow thrill over it is still present after the ligatures are tied.

The ligation technique of closure should only be used when the PDA is longer than it is wide, when it is not calcified and when the PDA is not infected. The ligature material should be relatively thick in order to avoid 'cutting' the tissue and two ligatures should be applied firmly. The best way of ensuring a safe closure of the PDA is to cross-clamp the proximal aorta for a few seconds before tying the ligatures. This causes the PDA to become flaccid and easier to ligate (Fig. 9.2).

The PDA should be divided between clamps if it is wider than it is long. Again, for the short time which it is necessary to do this, temporary cross-clamping of the proximal aorta will ensure that the aortic clamp does not slip off. The PDA should be half divided and that incision sewn up before the division is completed (Fig. 9.3). This manoeuvre ensures that an accident with a clamp would lead to a less severe haemorrhage.

If the PDA is calcified or infected, it will certainly need dividing. Placing a clamp on the aortic end of such a PDA is likely to rupture the diseased structure; the aorta must therefore be controlled above and below the ductus and a clamp placed on the extreme pulmonary artery end of the PDA before it is divided. Depending on the skill of the surgeon and the speed at which he can do this, the need may arise to preserve the spinal cord and kidneys with some form of left heart bypass.

Injury to the PDA during ligation or division

If ligatures are applied too tightly to a PDA under aortic pressure, there is likely to be some damage to the wall of the PDA. If this is severe, there will be obvious haemorrhage. If less severe, the ensuing weakness may dilate and form an aneurysm later. The technique of cross-clamping the proximal aorta during ligation has done much to reduce the incidence of this complication but care is still needed when applying tension during tying of the ligatures. If there is no haemorrhage, obviously no change has been effected, but the development of a false aneurysm should

Table 9.1
Complications of closure of PDA.

1 Failure to close the PDA
2 Injury to the PDA during ligation or division
3 Injury to adjacent structures
4 Inappropriate surgery for the condition

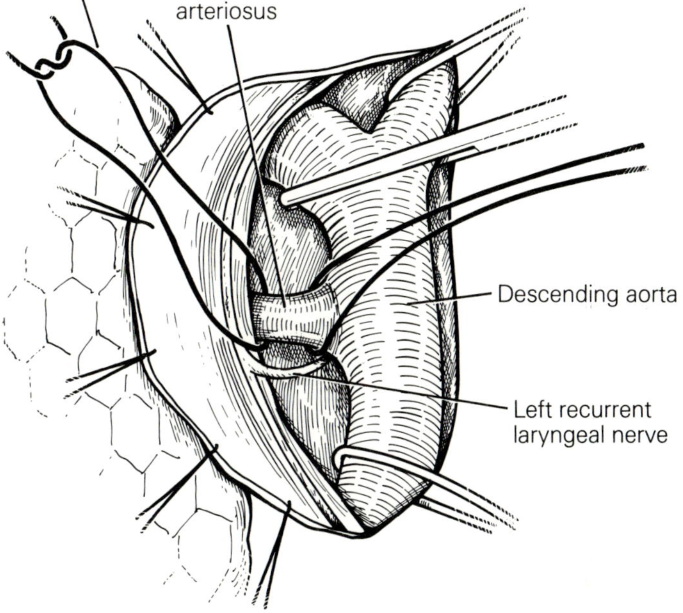

Figure 9.2 One method of ligation of the persistent ductus arteriosus.

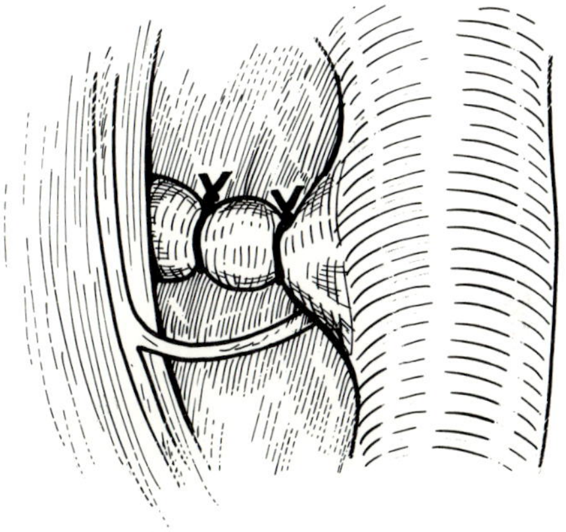

be excluded by chest X-rays when the patient is seen for follow up after surgery.

Damage to the PDA during division occurs as a result of applying the clamp at its aortic end to calcified or infected tissue. The operating surgeon should therefore gently palpate the PDA before applying clamps. Any suggestion of an abnormality should lead to the aortic end of the PDA being controlled by clamps on the aorta above and below the site. If in spite of all precautions

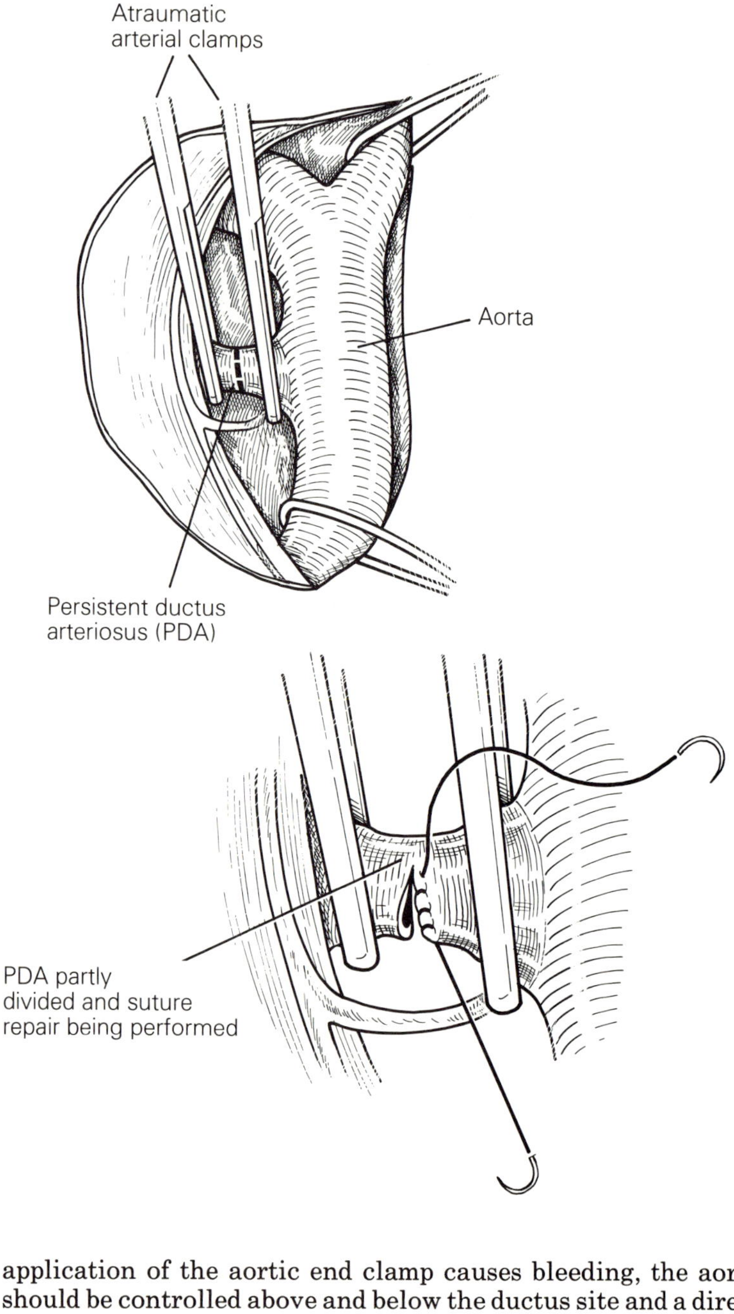

Figure 9.3
One method of dividing the persistent ductus arteriosus.

application of the aortic end clamp causes bleeding, the aorta should be controlled above and below the ductus site and a direct repair made of the laceration.

The need for emergency control of the aorta may arise without warning even if great care has been taken. For this reason, it is the routine to place tapes around the aorta before starting to dissect out the PDA.

Injury to adjacent structures

The aorta. This is dealt with on the lines suggested above.

The pulmonary artery. Haemorrhage from the pulmonary artery end of the PDA is rare because of the lower pressures involved. Should it occur, however, it is easily repaired with the intermittent use of the finger to control haemorrhage. Buttressed sutures will usually be needed to avoid tearing the tissue.

The left recurrent laryngeal nerve. This structure can usually be identified as it curves round the lower aspect of the PDA but some 3–4 mm away from it, closely applied to the mediastinal pleura (see Fig. 9.2). Once identified, the subsequent manoeuvres are carried out well away from it.

The thoracic duct. This structure crosses anteriorly from right to left of the body of the fourth thoracic vertebra. Occasionally it is damaged during operations in this region, such as repair of a coarctation of the aorta or closure of a PDA. The damage may be seen at the time of operation as a persisting leak of chyle is sucked away. The source is carefully identified and controlled with a transfixion stitch. Diathermy causes temporary control only.

After the operation, damage to the thoracic duct should be suspected if there is a continuing leak of clear fluid from the chest drain. Laboratory examination of this will confirm its origin. Most chylous-fistula leaks rapidly reduce in volume and stop altogether within a few days. Therefore, an expectant management is justified for a while, but if after a few days the discharge has not greatly diminished, the leak will need further surgery to stop it. The patient with a persisting chylous leak will tend to lose weight rapidly and this is another reason for early operative intervention.

Lymphangiograms are unnecessary in this condition as the site of the injury is known.

Before the operation, the patient is given several sandwiches, the butter in which has been stained with a fat-soluble dye. This renders identification of the thoracic duct, proximal to the lesion and in the right chest, very easy indeed. The right chest is opened and the tissues anterior to and to the right of the seventh and eighth thoracic vertebrae dissected. The thoracic duct is easily identified and doubly ligated with non-absorbing material.

Inappropriate surgery for the condition

The excessive flow through the lungs as a result of the PDA may cause hypertrophic and obliterative changes in the small pulmonary vessels. The resistance to flow rises and may exceed the systemic resistance. When that happens, the flow of blood through the ductus will reverse and the patient will become cyanosed. This process of reversal of a left-to-right shunt as a result of pulmonary vascular disease is known as the Eisenmenger reaction.

In those unfortunate patients with PDA who develop the Eisenmenger reaction, the flow of blood from the right ventricle becomes more and more dependent upon the presence of the PDA. Its ligation at this stage will lead to the death of the patient from right heart obstruction.

Obviously, no surgeon is going to operate on a patient with PDA and an established Eisenmenger reaction. But there are some patients, perhaps those with a reactive pulmonary tree, in whom it is not possible to say with complete confidence that the reaction is present. These patients are submitted to surgery to try and avoid their progressing to that stage. When such patients are operated on, it is wise to occlude the PDA temporarily, say for five to ten minutes, before deciding whether the patient will benefit.

Coarctation of the aorta

This condition accounts for some 10% of congenital cardiac lesions. It consists of a shelf-like obstruction in the aorta – usually just distal to the origin of the left subclavian artery – which impedes the flow of blood (Fig. 9.4). Both from the obstruction and from the activation of the renin–angiotensin mechanism in the kidneys, the systemic arterial pressure rises and will shorten the patient's life. Infection may occur on the coarctation and spontaneous dissection of the aorta may happen. The condition is associated with abnormalities of the aortic valve and with intracranial aneurysms.

Removal of the coarctation is performed to prevent these complications (Fig. 9.5). It is a 'closed' procedure and carries specific complications (Table 9.2).

Preoperative management. The site of the coarctation should be identified by angiography so that the surgical approach can be planned accordingly. The coarctation should not be assumed to be in the common site – angiography will show the location of the abnormality and also any aneurysmal intercostal arteries.

Haemorrhage

The chest wall contains the collateral circulation which develops as a result of the aortic obstruction. The increased vascularity causes excessive bleeding during the approach to the coarctation by left thoracotomy. Painstaking control of all blood vessels is necessary and each vessel should be ligated. Failure to ensure adequate control at this point will lead to persisting bleeding which may kill the patient if severe and at best will cause morbidity from a wound haematoma afterwards. An enlarged vessel may be damaged as the chest drain is inserted and the site of chest drainage must be inspected to ensure this complication has not occurred.

The intercostal arteries may be particularly troublesome. Close to the coarctation site, they may become paper thin and aneurysmal with a considerable flow of blood through them.

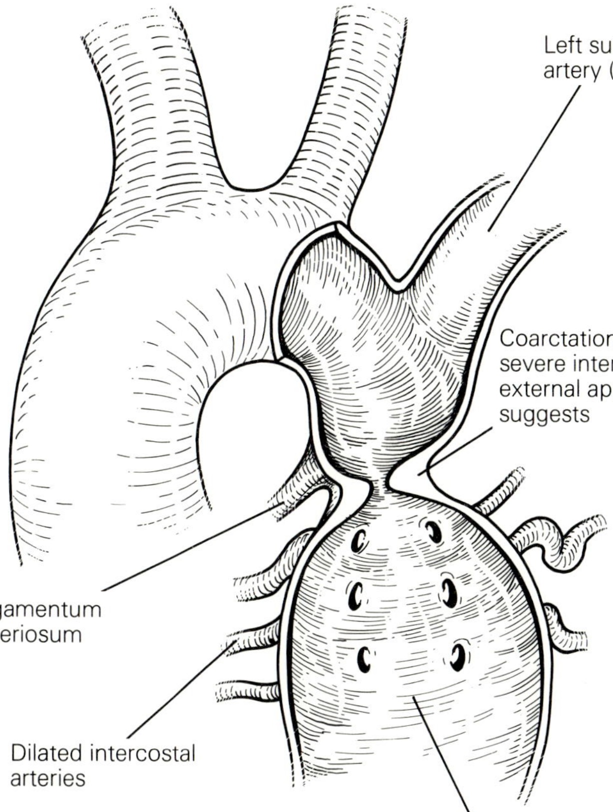

Figure 9.4 Anatomy of coarctation of the aorta in its most common position.

Again, painstaking dissection and control is necessary especially of those on the right side of the aorta. No more than one or two are normally divided because of the dangers to the spinal cord (see below).

The major danger of haemorrhage arises from the aorta. When the aorta above and below the coarctation is controlled, the coarctation is usually excised. Continuity of the aorta is re-established either by direct anastomosis or the insertion of a short segment of synthetic graft. Occasionally, the coarctation is not removed but merely opened and an onlay graft patch sewn into position as a gusset. In any event, the tissues are thin and the suture line is required to take a high pressure. A high degree of skill is required to achieve safe suture lines. The efficiency of the suture line is usually apparent in the operating room. Extra sutures may be needed to control individual bleeding points.

After the operation, the chest drains will indicate if blood is being lost externally and chest X-ray will show any intrathoracic

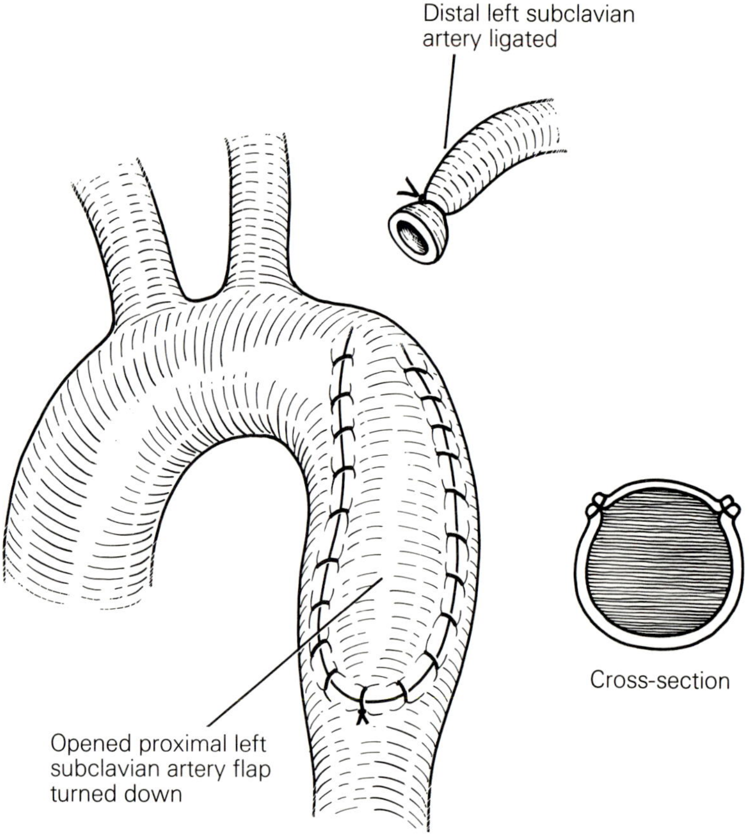

Figure 9.5 Principle of the subclavian flap operation in the correction of coarctation of the aorta in infants and young children.

Table 9.2 Complications of resection of coarctation of the aorta.

1 Haemorrhage
  (a) From the chest wall
  (b) From the intercostal arteries
  (c) From the aorta
2 Injury to the left recurrent laryngeal nerve and the thoracic duct
3 Spinal cord ischaemic necrosis leading to paraplegia
4 Mesenteric arteritis
5 Recurrence

accumulations. Usually bleeding will cease within 12 hours, but the drains are left in position for at least 36 hours. Bleeding may persist and in these cases the chest should be re-explored in the operating theatre. Very rarely, and usually as the result of a surge of blood pressure ripping a barely adequate suture line, there may be a catastrophic loss of blood from the aorta leading to cardiac arrest. This desperate situation may be relieved by rapidly opening the chest in the intensive care ward and stopping the bleeding by pressure.

Injury to the left recurrent laryngeal nerve and thoracic duct

These complications are discussed on page 179.

Spinal cord injury

The blood supply to the spinal cord is variable. Usually, there is an anterior spinal artery which runs longitudinally along the thoracic part of the spinal cord and this takes its supply from the intercostal arteries as it passes downwards. Occasionally, however, one or more of the intercostal arteries may be functional 'end' arteries and may thus be the sole supply of one segment of the spinal cord. Interruption of these will cause ischaemic necrosis of the segment and lead to paraplegia. This complication may occur because one or more intercostal arteries near to the coarctation site may need to be ligated in order to gain control of the blood flow in the aorta, permitting resection of the coarctation. A less common cause of spinal cord damage occurs when the surgeon operates on a coarctation with a poorly developed collateral circulation. Clamping the aorta may lead to distal ischaemia and the possibility of spinal cord damage. This possibility may be avoided by operating only on those cases of coarctation which are truly obstructive, i.e. those which are associated with upper limb hypertension, absent or delayed femoral pulses and a well-developed collateral circulation in the chest wall. In these circumstances, the distal aorta retains a high pressure when the aorta clamps are applied. Should the distal aortic pressure fall very much when the coarctation is clamped, serious doubts about the wisdom of resecting the abnormality should be felt.

Most cases of paraplegia after resection of coarctation are due to the interruption of an intercostal artery which is an end artery to one segment of the spinal cord. The complication is largely prevented by restricting the number of intercostal arteries which are ligated to one or perhaps two. However, this disastrous complication is unpredictable even with that precaution. All patients about to have the operation should be aware of this remote possibility.

Mesenteric arteritis

This is also a rare but troublesome complication of coarctation resection and is caused by a reactive arteriolar spasm in the mesenteric circulation which occurs after the operation. The cause of the spasm is not known, but is most likely due to a response to the normal flow of blood so long denied by the presence of the aortic obstruction. The result of the spasm is ischaemia of a greater or lesser part of the gut and sometimes necrosis. The amount of necrosis may be large, in which case the patient's life will be in danger.

This complication is preventable by the means of controlling the arterial pressure after operation within the normal range by the liberal use of hypotensive agents. Certainly, any rise of the arterial systolic pressure above 140 mmHg should be treated.

Any patient who complains of abdominal pain after resection of coarctation of the aorta should be managed as an early acute abdominal emergency. Certainly, the cause of the discomfort should not be assumed to be mesenteric arteritis; the author removed an acutely inflamed appendix in one child three days after a coarctation operation.

Recurrence

As coarctation is diagnosed earlier and earlier, so smaller children present for its correction. In infants the aorta is small, and if the coarctation is resected and an aortic end-to-end anastomosis done, this anastomosis will usually fail to grow no matter what sewing technique is used. Recurrence of obstruction will inevitably occur and lead to a further operation which may be technically difficult and hazardous for the patient.

In infants and small children, resection of the coarctation and end-to-end anastomosis should be avoided. Instead the coarctation is opened longitudinally and a flap of living tissue inserted as a gusset, thus abolishing the obstruction. The flap is obtained by turning down and opening the divided left subclavian artery.

Recurrence of coarctation may occur in larger individuals as a result of an imperfect technique of end-to-end repair. Many surgeons have used a prosthetic patch to abolish the coarctation obstruction as in younger children.

Shunt operations in congenital heart disease

Many simple and complex congenital abnormalities may cause an impaired blood flow to the lungs and thus impair oxygenation. Such abnormalities include pulmonary stenosis, tricuspid atresia and tetralogy of Fallot. As a consequence of the impaired oxygenation the child is cyanosed, causing a range of symptoms such as tiredness, poor growth and abnormalities such as polycythaemia.

Ideally, of course, such anatomical lesions should be corrected at an early age, but often the anatomy is unsuitable for early correction of the child too sick to withstand a prolonged operation. Palliation can be achieved by operations which increase the pulmonary blood flow by directing blood into the pulmonary circulation by a 'shunt'. There are several types of shunt:

1 Subclavian artery to pulmonary artery (Blalock–Taussig) (Fig. 9.6).
2 Descending aorta to pulmonary artery (Potts) (Fig. 9.7).
3 Ascending aorta to pulmonary artery (Waterston) (Fig. 9.8).
4 Superior vena cava to pulmonary artery (Glenn).

Complications of shunt operations

Shunt is too small. This situation arises as a result of technical problems encountered in operation on these small children. The

Figure 9.6
Blalock–Taussig shunt.

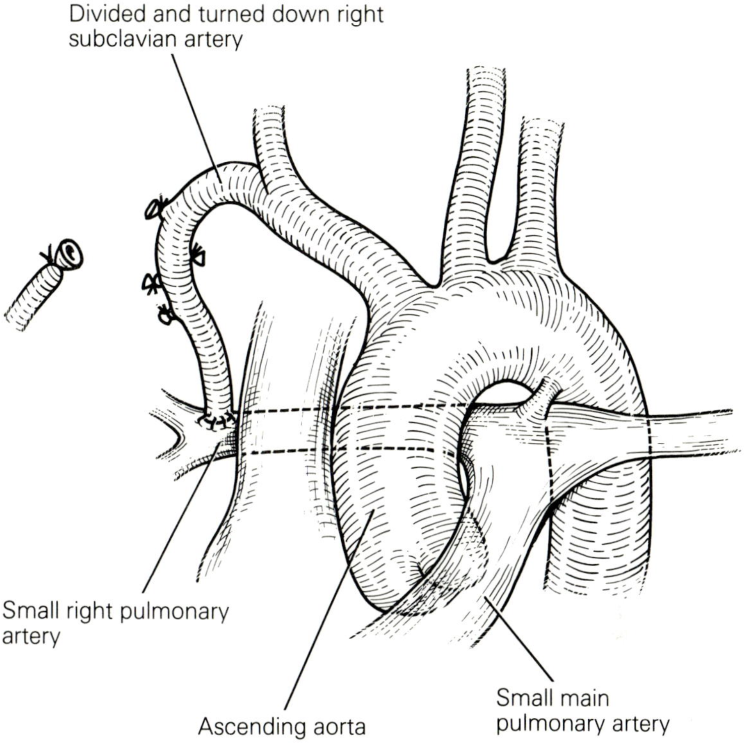

Figure 9.7
Potts' shunt.

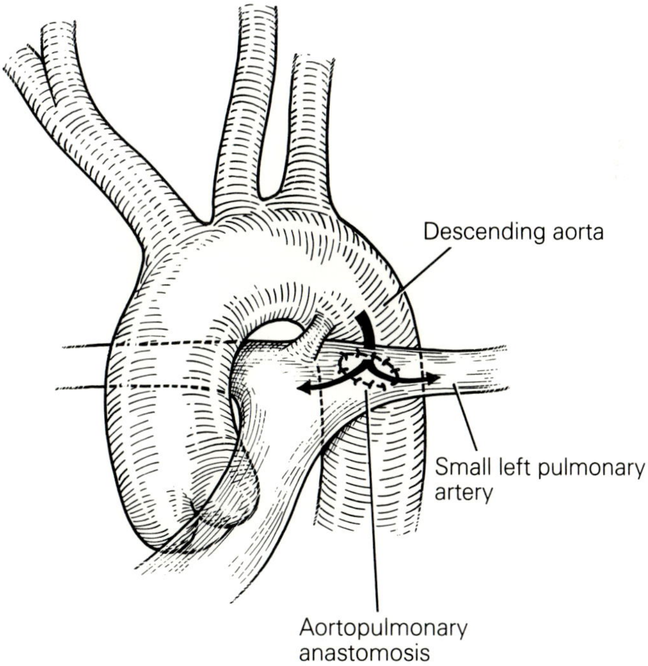

Figure 9.8
Waterston shunt.

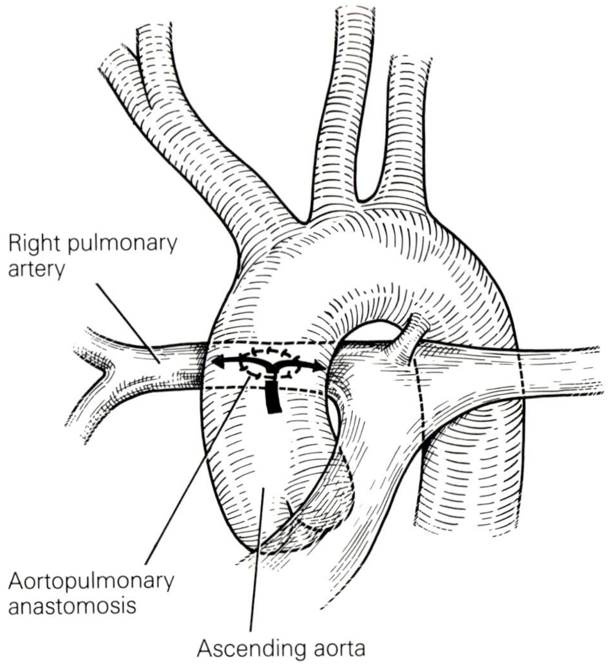

shunt anastomosis may be difficult to see but optical magnification will help. Interrupted rather than continuous sutures will avoid further narrowing of a small anastomosis. An inadequate shunt will usually thrombose.

Shunt is too large. If an excessive volume of blood passes into the pulmonary circulation, then the left heart may be placed under strain and may fail (except in the Glenn operation). In addition, the excessive flow of blood into the lungs may cause oedema in the immediate postoperative period and later obliterative pulmonary vascular disease may develop leading to the Eisenmenger syndrome.

Calculation of the size of the shunt is therefore a matter of considerable judgement. In neonates and small infants a shunt of 3 mm in diameter is about right, but later up to 5 mm may be needed.

Summary

Closed operations for congenital heart disease may be corrective (as in the closure of persistent ductus arteriosus and correction of coarctation of the aorta), or palliative as in the creation of a shunt. Closed corrective operations are ideally performed in the first two years of life. Shunt operations are a prelude to corrective surgery. Since correction is performed at an earlier age, shunt operations are being done less frequently. Judging the correct size of a shunt is difficult and specific problems will occur if the shunt is too large or too small.

Persisting controversies

- Should the PDA be ligated or divided?
- Should coarctation be excised or treated by an onlay flap?
- The most suitable shunting procedure.

Complications of Open-Heart Surgery for Congenital Heart Disease

Open-heart surgery for congenital heart disease is being offered to younger and younger patients. The number of children being operated on in the first year of life is growing as experience and techniques progressively reduce the risks. As stated previously, the advantages of early correction to the patient are very great and as long as the operation can be performed safely, early surgery will occur increasingly frequently.

Although the principles of the operations remain the same as in older age groups, the small size and often specific physiological requirements of these small children make the area highly specialized. This group of patients is therefore best served by a paediatric cardiac surgical team which is totally committed and experienced.

The complications which may arise from the perioperative management of these children are many and often specific to the somewhat uncommon lesions which are to be corrected (Table 9.3). As such they are beyond the scope of this chapter. However, certain broad groups of complications may be identified and these will be described.

Problems relating to size

Increasingly complex procedures are being performed as open operations on increasingly small children. Most surgeons operating on small children find that some form of simple optical magnification is necessary to ensure a precise operation. The magnification is usually 2–4 × and several varieties of magnifying spectacles are available commercially.

Access is usually achieved via a median sternotomy. The supple nature of the chest wall allows wide retraction and gives good exposure of all parts of the heart.

Table 9.3
Specific problems of open-heart surgery in children.

1 Size
2 Physiological requirements of small children
3 Bleeding
4 Pulmonary problems
5 Conduction problems

Cannulas for cardiopulmonary bypass and most of the surgical instruments should be appropriately small sized. Metallic rather than plastic cannulas are used in the cannulation of the aorta because of their improved internal diameter. The bypass technique is modified in small children by the addition of extreme hypothermia (16–20 °C). At this temperature, the circulation may be safely arrested for up to one hour and even the most complex problems can be repaired in this time. Recently, some evidence of neuronal damage in experimental animals has been produced as an argument against this technique and there is a tendency for full flow bypass with moderate hypothermia to be performed, as in the adult. Minor neuronal damage is very difficult to detect and may be shown only much later by a failure of intellectual development.

The small body weight means a relatively low thermal capacity and this, coupled with rather insensitive temperature control, means that infants can easily become hypothermic during the operation or afterwards. Hence the need for warm operating rooms and warming water blankets under each patient.

The low body weight indicates a low blood volume and the use of haemodilution is much more restricted during cardiopulmonary bypass. Usually, some donor blood is needed to maintain the packed cell volume at the acceptable level of 25% and this blood should not be more than three days old. Many surgeons insist on fresh blood throughout the operation.

Problems due to specific physiological requirements of small children

Fluid replacement and loss are critical at much smaller volumes than in the adult and gross derangements can arise quite quickly. The 24-hour fluid balance chart is too unresponsive to rapid changes and a six-hourly chart is more appropriate. Infants tend to lose fluid by the insensible route more easily than adults, and their metabolic rate may be up to three times that of the normal adult. The maintenance fluid requirement is around 80 ml/kg body weight $\cdot$ 24 h^{-1} but in infants under 10 kg, 100 ml/kg $\cdot$ 24 h^{-1} is required.

Specific electrolyte derangements are frequently encountered. Frequently, hypernatraemia may result from excessive saline infusion or from sodium bicarbonate being used to correct acidosis. The calcium level is very labile, needing frequent monitoring and correction if necessary. Similarly, the glucose level may vary enormously and needs similar attention.

The kidneys and liver of small children are immature enzymatically. The kidneys are less capable to deal with a solute load or acidosis than those of the adult. Certain liver enzyme systems, notably the glycerol transference system, are similarly deficient and unable to handle some drugs.

Nutrition is essential because of the high metabolic rate of these children. Usually their recovery permits eating within one or two days, but if normal feeding is not established by that time, enteral (or, exceptionally, parenteral) nutrition should be started.

The precise monitoring and management of all these physiological problems involves considerable paediatric experience and knowledge and are therefore best left entirely to the paediatrician on the team.

Bleeding

Small volumes of blood loss rapidly become significant in the small child and are managed by infusion of blood to maintain a satisfactory left or right atrial pressure. As in the adult, surgical haemostasis is of cardinal importance. As stated before, most paediatric cardiac surgeons are in favour of using fresh blood for children because of its oxygen carrying superiority and because fresh blood contains all the labile elements of clotting (some perhaps as yet undescribed) which promote sound haemostasis. The need for detailed coagulation studies is less important than in adults, if that were possible.

Excessive bleeding should always lead to early exploration as in the adult, but the level at which bleeding becomes excessive will vary with the child's size and with the surgeon's temperament.

Pulmonary problems

Infants and small children have many pulmonary complications after cardiac surgery and these are due to the following three groups of causes, either singly or in combination.

The small calibre of the airways makes collapse and atelectasis very common, and yet very difficult to treat. Instrumentation carries the risk of provoking oedema which further increases the hazards. Frequent careful physiotherapy and suction will reduce this complication. Mucolytic agents, such as normal saline or *N*-acetylcysteine, will prevent mucous plugs forming.

The pulmonary vasculature. This circulation is very labile. Acidosis and an increased level of carbon dioxide in the arterial blood will cause intense vasoconstriction even in 'normal' pulmonary vessels. In those cardiac abnormalities which lead to an excessive flow of blood to the lungs (the left-to-right shunts), further changes may occur.

At birth, the pulmonary arterial tree consists of vessels with the same thickness and characteristics as the systemic arteries. Normally, there is a progressive loss of wall thickness by a process of involution, producing the rather thin-walled pulmonary vessels. This process is usually completed by the third year of life. In conditions such as ventricular septal defect, where there is excessive pulmonary blood flow from the beginning, this involution does not occur and the embryonic wall thickness persists. Later, medial and intimal hypertrophy occurs and gradually the lumen of the pulmonary arteries is reduced. At first there is a considerable element of spasm, but later the lumen is reduced by permanent wall changes which are irreversible.

Physiologically, the resistance to flow within the pulmonary circulation begins to rise and eventually reaches systemic levels and above, at which time the original left-to-right shunt reverses and the child becomes cyanosed. This is called the Eisenmenger reaction (see above, page 179).

Surgical correction of cardiac lesions which are causing excessive pulmonary blood flow can only be performed when the pulmonary resistance is less than systemic. As the level of the pulmonary resistance increases, so do the risks of the operation. This is another reason why surgery on lesions such as ventricular septal defect and persistent ductus arteriosus is performed at an early stage.

Poor resistance to infection. Contamination by organisms of the bronchial tree leads to infection of the pulmonary parenchyma very readily in the small child. With the small calibre of the bronchial tree, the infection tends to be more resistant to antibiotic treatment than might be expected. Meticulous aseptic techniques of endotracheal suction will help to reduce the frequency of contamination. Frequent bacteriological testing of the sputum is necessary. Once infection is established, antibiotics are given according to the sensitivities of the organisms identified, *but* frequent physiotherapy and humidification are equally important.

Conduction problems

Many of the lesions correctable by surgery are closely related to the conduction mechanisms of the heart. For instance, the bundle of His runs very close to the posterior and inferior margins of a ventricular septal defect and the atrioventricular node is in danger when any atrioventricular defect is repaired. Although the course of the conducting pathways is known in most cases, there remain a number of patients with extremely complex lesions or with abnormally sited conducting pathways in whom surgery may damage conduction. The usual result of this is atrioventricular block which results in a slow ventricular rate and an inadequate cardiac output.

Every effort should be made at the time of operation to avoid the conducting tissue. At the conclusion of the operation, epicardial pacing wires are placed on the ventricles and atria and brought out through the skin. If needed, external pacing can be achieved by these; if they are not needed, they may be removed by traction at 7–10 days after surgery.

Summary

Open-heart surgery in infants and small children is being practised at increasingly younger ages. Small children have specific problems in addition to those common to all open-heart operations and cardiopulmonary bypass procedures. The major areas for concern arise as a result of low body weight and specific physiological requirements. Bleeding, pulmonary and conduction problems are common. The care of these small children should be supervised by a paediatrician and the surgeon. Emphasis is placed on the rapidity of changes which might occur, and the need for close observation and monitoring.

Complications of Some Common Open-Heart Operations in Children

Atrial septal defect

Defects in the formation of the atrial septum situated anteriorly to the ostium of the coronary sinus are 'primum' defects and those situated posteriorly to the coronary sinus are 'secundum' defects (Fig. 9.9). The essential difference is that primum defects are always associated with some abnormality of the mitral or tricuspid valve and that surgical closure may damage the atrioventricular (AV) node. Secundum defects, on the other hand, are not related to the conduction mechanism and there are no related abnormalities of the atrioventricular valves.

Closure of a secundum defect under open-heart conditions is one of the safest operations in cardiac surgery. Those dangers that do exist, however, stem from the need for cardiopulmonary bypass and the dangers of air embolism. The actual closure of the secundum defect may not be sound, unless the actual edges of the defect are firmly apposed. Accurate identification of the margins may be made difficult by thin endocardial curtains partially closing the defect and which, if sewn, provide very weak closure.

The eustachian valve at the entry of the inferior vena cava into the right atrium may be incorporated in the repair unless a specific manoeuvre (see Fig. 9.9) is used. If the eustachian valve is sewn into the repair, blood from the inferior vena cava can pass into the left atrium and cause deep cyanosis.

Secundum defects high in the atrial septum (the so-called sinus venosus defects) should always be patched using pericardium because direct suture repair may constrict the entry of the superior vena cava into the right atrium. Sinus venosus defects are frequently associated with a pulmonary vein from the right lung draining into the superior vena cava rather than the left atrium. This vein is usually left since it carries only a small amount of blood.

After surgery, very few specific complications arise. An increased incidence of supraventricular tachycardia has been noted.

Closure of primum atrial septal defects is always achieved by the use of a patch in order to avoid distortion of the atrioventricular valves. Abnormalities of the valves are usually corrected at the same operation.

Figure 9.9
Anatomy of an atrial septal defect of the secundum type.

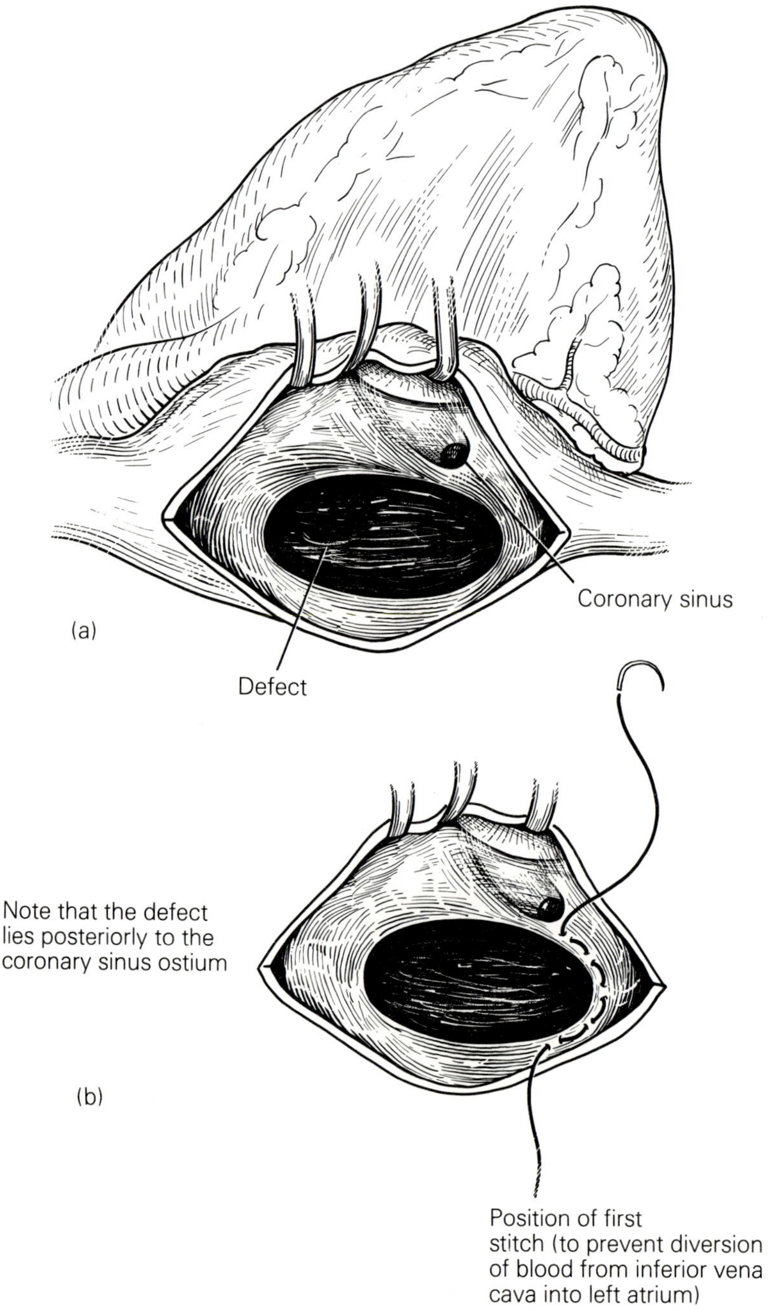

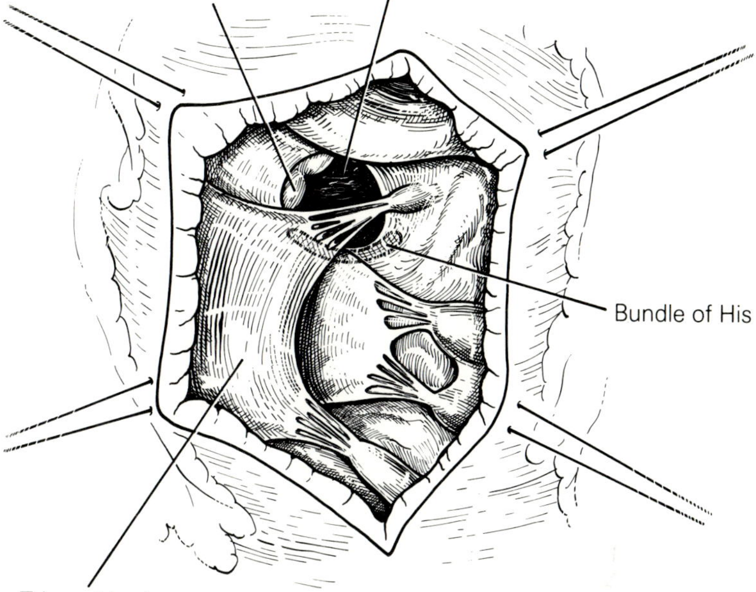

Figure 9.10 Anatomy of the ventricular septal defect of the infracristal type.

Damage to the AV node and the bundle of His is avoided by the use of multiple interrupted sutures inserted precisely into the exact edge of the defect or by placing the patch to the right hand side of the coronary sinus ostium thus avoiding the danger area altogether.

Summary Atrial septal defects are of the secundum or the primum type depending on their relationship to the ostium of the coronary sinus. Secundum defects are easily closed, but closure of primum defects is more difficult because of the possibility of damage to the conduction system or to the atrioventricular valves.

Persisting controversy

- Patch closure or direct closure of secundum atrial septal defect.

Ventricular septal defect

Ventricular septal defects (VSD) may occur in any part of the interventricular septum. They may be subpulmonary (type I); related to the tricuspid valve (type II); or situated in the muscular septum (type III). The type II VSD is most common and is closely related to the bundle of His. Ventricular septal defects are usually single, but may be multiple.

Closure is advised in all defects if the pulmonary flow is twice that of the systemic circulation. Because of the possibility of pulmonary vascular damage early closure is performed. Closure is usually achieved by patching, using synthetic fabric. There are many techniques used, reflecting the lack of any one wholly suitable method.

The principal hazards are:

1 Inadequate closure.
2 Damage to the bundle of His.
3 Damage to other structures.

Inadequate closure. There is normally a considerable difference of pressure between the right and left ventricles and this places stress on the repair of a VSD. All sutures should be placed accurately around the edges of the defect. Some surgeons use a continuous suture, but most use multiple buttressed sutures.

Damage to the bundle of His (Fig. 9.10). In the type II defect, the bundle of His lies to the posteroinferior quadrant of the defect and about 3 mm from its margin. Sutures must therefore be placed either in the exact margin of the defect or about 7 mm away, in which case they are inserted into the medial part of the tricuspid valve ring.

Damage to other structures. This danger is most commonly encountered in the repair of a type II defect, which is related not only to the tricuspid valve but more importantly to the aortic valve. Accurate placement of the suture is helped by the use of cardioplegia which gives a flaccid, quiet, bloodless heart.

Summary

The complications of VSD closure are due to:

1 Imperfect closure (?more than one defect).
2 Damage to the bundle of His.
3 Damage to adjacent structures.

If the operation is successfully accomplished, however, the degree of damage to the pulmonary circulation is the major risk factor.

Persisting controversy

- At what level of pulmonary vascular damage is closure of the VSD impossible?

Pulmonary valve stenosis

Failure of the cusps of the pulmonary valve to develop as separate structures results in an obstruction to the flow of blood from the right ventricle into the pulmonary artery. Hypertrophy of the right ventricle and a poor pulmonary blood flow follow. The pressure load arising as a result of the obstruction leads to a tendency towards sudden deterioration of right ventricular function and death. Any obstruction within the heart leads to similar sudden and catastrophic results.

The surgical relief of the obstruction leads to immediate

improvement in both pulmonary blood flow and in right ventricular function. The operation is performed under open conditions through the pulmonary artery. The fused commissures of the valve are opened and separated from the wall of the artery. Provided the obstruction is relieved, there are no complications to this operation. However, if any residual obstruction remains, severe cardiac failure can result.

This lesion is described not because of its frequent occurrence, but because it illustrates the general principle that the relief of intracardiac obstruction is a major objective of cardiac surgery, whether the obstruction lies in the chambers, the valves or the great vessels of the heart. Failure to relieve fully the obstruction is the major complication of such operations. At operation, pressure measurements upstream and downstream of the obstruction will show the degree of relief obtained. Pressure differences of more than 50 mmHg usually indicate severe obstruction.

Summary The relief of obstruction within the heart will confer major benefits whereas the failure to abolish it will cause severe postoperative problems. Pulmonary valve stenosis represents one condition which is obstructive, but any unrelieved obstruction within the heart or great vessels is very dangerous.

Tetralogy of Fallot

This is the most common combination of lesions causing cyanosis. The major abnormalities are a ventricular septal defect and an obstruction to the outflow of the right ventricle. As a result of these, hypertrophy of the right ventricle and a very large aorta 'overriding' the ventricular septal defect complete the tetrad. This condition is described because it is very common and because the combination of a shunt and an obstruction lead to predictable consequences.

As a result of the obstruction to outflow from the right ventricle, the pressure in the right ventricle rises and exceeds the pressure in the left. As a result, a right-to-left shunt of deoxygenated blood occurs, resulting in desaturation of the arterial blood. The patient becomes cyanosed and has a poor exercise tolerance. The poor pulmonary blood flow is another major cause of desaturation. The surgical treatment of congenital cardiac disease began with this disease when Blalock devised the shunt which bears his name. However, the total correction of the obstruction and intracardiac shunt is now practised widely.

The complications of the operation which are specific arise from two sources:

1 Failure to close the shunt.
2 Failure to relieve the obstruction.

Failure to close the shunt. The VSD in tetralogy of Fallot is large and situated close to the aortic and tricuspid valves. Apart from its size, the complications which might occur are those of any other simple VSD, with the possible exception that in the tetralogy of Fallot the bundle of His is less likely to be damaged.

Failure to relieve the obstruction. The obstruction in tetralogy of Fallot may lie at the ring of the pulmonary valve or above or below it. The latter arises as a result of hypertrophy in the muscle bands of the infundibulum or outflow of the right ventricle. Analysis of surgical results shows clearly that the mortality after total correction of the tetralogy of Fallot is related to the degree of obstruction left at the end of the operation. With this in mind, the operating surgeon may merely excise muscle or place a large patch across the outflow of the right ventricle, or even insert an artificial conduit between the right ventricle and the distal main pulmonary artery.

Summary The tetralogy of Fallot illustrates the general principle that the outcome of a congenital cardiac operation is mainly determined by the quality of the repair performed in the operating room. As long as no myocardial damage is inflicted in the process, the secure closure of defects and the abolition of obstruction will lead to good cardiac function and survival. Failure to achieve these two objectives usually causes problems which even the most expert postoperative care may not be able to overcome. The general complications of cardiopulmonary bypass and of open-heart surgery may still happen, of course, but are of secondary importance to these two major complications.

Conclusion

The variety and complexity of the many congenital abnormalities affecting the heart is beyond the scope of this volume. Detailed description of individual lesions is to be found in major texts devoted to the subject. The abnormalities described in this section have been chosen in order to represent the types of anomaly which may occur and the complications which may follow.

In congenital cardiac surgery, all other factors being equal, the prime determinants of success are the quality of the correction and the quality of the myocardial protection. Both of these lie within the control of the operating surgeon and fine details of technique are important. The special needs of infants and small children in the pre- and postoperative periods have to be met; the best way of looking after such patients is by a joint anaesthetic, paediatric and surgical team, together with appropriately trained nurses and technical staff. With such a combination of expertise, smaller and younger children may be operated on with success and with considerable advantages to their future development and well-being.

Further reading

Barratt Boyes, B.G., Neutze, J.M. & Harris, E.A. (1973) *Heart Disease in Infancy*. Edinburgh and London: Churchill Livingstone.

Blalock, A. (1946) Operative closure of the patent ductus arteriosus. *Surg. Gynecol. Obstet.*, *82*, 113.

Crafoord, C. & Nylin, G. (1945) Congenital coarctation of the aorta and its treatment. *J. Thorac. Surg.*, *14*, 347.

Dillard, D.H., Mohri, H. & Merendino, K.A. (1974) Correction of heart disease in infancy using deep hypothermia with total circulatory arrest. *J. Thorac. Cardiovasc. Surg.*, *61*, 589.

Keith, J.D., Rowe, R.D. & Vlad, P. (1958) *Heart Disease in Infancy and Childhood*. New York: Macmillan.

Kirklin, J.W. & Karp, R.B. (1970) *Tetralogy of Fallot from a Surgical Viewpoint*. Philadelphia: W.B. Saunders.

Tawes, R.L., Bull, J.C. & Rose, B.B. (1970) Hypertension and abdominal pain after resection of aortic coarctation. *Ann. Surg.*, *171*, 409.

10 Complications of Surgery on the Thoracic Aorta

The thoracic aorta is a large structure and carries the whole of the cardiac output. Lesions of the aorta are always life threatening from the dangers of haemorrhage and damage to the viscera. The location of the lesions as well as their nature pose specific surgical problems and complications. Complications from bleeding are common after operation and are made worse by the need for cardiopulmonary bypass. Diseases affecting the ascending aorta, the arch and descending aorta will be considered separately as each part carries specific complications (Table 10.1).

Infection

Surgery to the thoracic aorta usually involves the insertion of a prosthetic graft. If this should become infected, the patient will almost certainly die of secondary haemorrhage. Replacement of the graft by a second graft may occasionally cure the infection. Antibiotic prophylaxis and a strictly aseptic technique are essential. Infection of a prosthesis in the aorta is a dreaded complication regarded by many surgeons as one of the few inoperable problems in cardiovascular surgery.

Surgery of the ascending aorta

The ascending aorta begins at the aortic ring and ends at the origin of the brachiocephalic or innominate artery. It has two major branches, the coronary arteries. Surgical isolation of the ascending aorta is possible only with the use of cardiopulmonary bypass. This technique is necessary in order to maintain the perfusion of all the body tissues during the procedure. The only tissue *not* perfused during operations on the ascending aorta is the myocardium. The surgeon operating on the ascending aorta must therefore use some form of myocardial preservation; at the time of writing, this is usually hyperkalaemic, hypothermic cardioplegia.

Cardiopulmonary bypass is of the conventional type used in open-heart surgery, with bicaval or right atrial cannulation for venous drainage and the arterial return is usually into the common femoral artery. Access to the ascending aorta is given by a median sternotomy and opening of the pericardium, as in cardiac surgery, and air embolism is an ever-present problem.

Surgery of the arch of the aorta

These operations also need cardiopulmonary bypass. The myocardium and the brain must also be protected during periods of

Table 10.1
Nature of lesions of the thoracic aorta.

1 *Ascending aorta*
Dissection
Ruptured sinus of Valsalva
Aneurysm
Annuloaortic ectasia
False aneurysm

2 *Arch of aorta*
Aneurysm
Traumatic avulsion of major branches

3 *Descending aorta*
Dissection
Coarctation
Aneurysm
Traumatic transection

isolation of the arch. As in the case of the myocardium, the method of cerebral protection depends on surgical experience and preference. Either perfusion of the carotid arteries or reduction in cerebral oxygen needs by hypothermia are possible. At the time of writing, the technical problems and inferior results of carotid perfusion have led to most surgeons relying on deep (15 °C) hypothermia and arrest of the cerebral circulation for up to 40 minutes as the preferred technique. Cardiopulmonary bypass is used in the same manner as in operations on the ascending aorta, but cooling to 15 °C is used. Cardioplegia and clamping of the carotid arteries is performed when the desired temperature is reached and the pump flow reduced to a very low level for the time it takes to carry out the surgical procedure on the arch.

Access is more difficult, but is usually adequate if a median sternotomy is extended to the left in its upper part. As with the ascending aorta, air embolism is a hazard.

Surgery of the descending aorta

Isolation of the descending aorta carries risks to the spinal cord and the abdominal viscera, especially the kidneys. Protection of the heart and the brain is not a problem since the heart can support a spontaneous circulation to these tissues. Some form of left heart bypass or perfusion to the lower trunk is essential. This may be done by one of the following methods:

1 Left atrial to femoral bypass.
2 Femoral vein to femoral artery bypass.
3 Ascending aorta to descending aorta shunt using a heparin-coated conduit (Gott Shunt).

Some experienced surgeons with superb speed take no measures at all to protect the spinal cord and lower body, but most surgeons will use one or other of the above techniques.

Access to the descending aorta is given by a full left thoracotomy. Anaesthesia for this should include a technique whereby the left lung can be collapsed, thus reducing the need for traction on it.

The thoracic duct and the left recurrent laryngeal nerve are both closely related to the descending aorta and both may be damaged during surgery. Damage to the spinal cord may occur in spite of a satisfactorily functioning perfusion technique. A major cause of such damage, which results in paraplegia, is a variation in the blood supply to the cord, particularly to its anterior columns. Normally, the anterior spinal artery is large and the segmental arteries make significant contributions to it. Sometimes, the anterior spinal artery is small and the blood supply to various levels of the cord is obtained from the segmental arteries. Depending on how much these arteries connect with each other, some may be functional end-arteries. Consequently some of the intercostal arteries coming off the ascending aorta may be the only vessels supplying that segment of the spinal cord and damage to the cord may arise unpredictably in operations on the descending aorta. Every patient should be warned of this before the operation.

Haemorrhage in Operations on the Thoracic Aorta

Severe bleeding is the most common fatal complication of all operations on the thoracic aorta. There are three major causes:

1 Imperfections of surgical technique.
2 Porous grafts.
3 Clotting abnormalities.

Imperfections of surgical technique

Most of the lesions requiring surgery are associated with either thin or unduly friable aortic walls and sometimes both. The high pressure within the aorta will impose a severe stress on such suture lines. The technique by which the anastomoses and repairs are performed needs to be perfect. Several specific points need stating:

1 The suture material should be a monofilament polypropylene material on an atraumatic needle (Prolene). This is used in a continuous manner and the very low friction of this material in the tissues leads to an evenly tensioned suture line.
2 A continuous everting suture technique is most effective. If the tissues are at all friable, this suturing technique may be made even safer by the use of Teflon felt buttresses.
3 The aorta being operated on is usually empty and without pressure. On the occasions when it is necessary to put stitches into the aorta which is carrying blood under pressure, that pressure should be momentarily reduced.

If the patient is on some form of partial or full cardiopulmonary bypass this is fairly easily done by reducing the flow into the patient for a short period. If there is no bypass in place, a short period of cross-clamping the inferior vena cava will predictably and safely lower the aortic pressure.

It is assumed that the needle and suture is passed through the aortic tissue in a manner which avoids tearing the tissue.

Porous grafts

Most thoracic aortic procedures involve the insertion of a synthetic fabric prosthesis. Whether this is knitted or woven in its manufacture, some bleeding will occur in the heparinized patient and this can be very troublesome. Preclotting of the graft may be performed by placing it in unheparinized blood until it clots. A more satisfactory procedure is to immerse the graft in a mixture of heparinized blood and normal saline and then to autoclave the graft for eight minutes. This results in a graft which is perfectly bloodtight. The use of diluted blood avoids the excessive deposition of altered blood which might fragment later and cause emboli.

Clotting abnormalities

Operations on the thoracic aorta tend to be prolonged and clotting abnormalities may arise. In addition, deep hypothermia as used in arch operations may further derange normal clotting. For these reasons, fresh blood should always be available in this type of operation.

Specific Problems of Operations on the Ascending Aorta

Dissection of the ascending aorta

The lesion is a transverse tear of the intima and media of the aorta occurring some 3 cm above the uppermost limit of the aortic valve. Blood is forced along a plane which separates the inner and outer media, and this plane of dissection may involve the whole of the aorta and its major branches. The suspensory mechanism of the aortic valve is lost and aortic regurgitation occurs. The pressure of blood in the false lumen may cause the thin outer layer to burst and this usually causes death by a bleed into the pericardium. The major branches of the aorta may be occluded by the pressure within the false lumen.

Dissection of the ascending aorta may be confirmed by angiography or by echocardiography. Once diagnosed, the dissection of the ascending aorta should be repaired because the prognosis without surgery, even if the aortic pressure is reduced by drugs, is very bad.

The aim of the operation is to remove the area which has torn and replace it with a prosthetic graft. This decompresses the false lumen. The aortic valve may be resuspended and rendered competent. The operation is performed under cardiopulmonary bypass and cardioplegia. The ascending aorta is clamped and opened. The tear is confirmed. The abnormal aorta is then excised and replaced with a 'cooked' prosthetic graft.

Complications

1 *Myocardial damage.* This is avoided by the use of cardioplegia.
2 *Cerebral damage.* This may be present before operation because of the effects of the false lumen on the cerebral vessels. A further cause is air from the opened aorta. A steep head-down tilt is recommended when the clamps are removed at the end of the repair.
3 *Bleeding.* If the suture technique used is as recommended above, the need for extra sutures is low and these may be inserted with safety, superficially to the original everting suture line.
4 *Haemopericardium.* This may occur as the patient is being prepared for surgery. The only hope in this desperate situation is to open the chest and control the bleeding by pressure until cardiopulmonary bypass can be instituted.
5 *Hypertension.* Hypertension after surgery should be vigorously controlled by vasodilators and β-blocking drugs.

In recent years, a rigid intraluminal graft has been introduced in order to simplify the operation (Fig. 10.1). This is inserted into the aorta and tapes used externally to fix it in place and stop bleeding. This innovation is most useful in dissections of the descending aorta but less so in those of the ascending aorta. The

Figure 10.1
Intraluminal aortic graft.

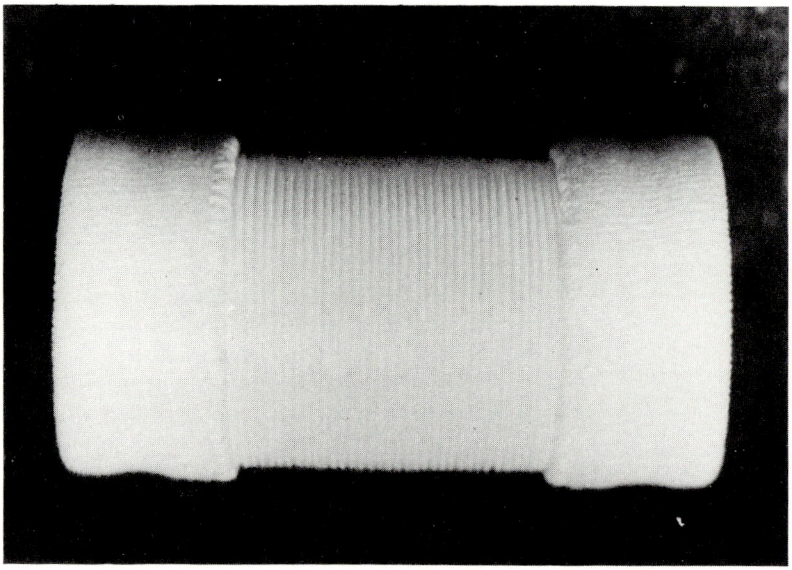

tear is often quite near to the aortic valve and it is difficult to site the prosthesis without interfering with the valve.

Ruptured sinus of Valsalva

This lesion is a congenital weakness of a sinus of Valsalva which gradually extends like a windsock and which may eventually penetrate and burst into any cardiac chamber. A large shunt from the ascending aorta to that cardiac chamber occurs. Diagnosis is made by aortography. The lesion should be closed at operation. The aortic end is usually situated just above a cusp of the aortic valve and is often near to the ostium of a coronary artery.

Damage to the valve or the coronary artery may be avoided by the careful insertion of a number of buttressed sutures. Otherwise the operation is not attended by any specific problems, although many prudent surgeons will close both ends of the lesion by opening the affected cardiac chamber.

Aneurysms of the ascending aorta

These may be localized or part of a general pathological dilatation of the aortic ring and ascending aorta (annuloaortic ectasis). The simple aneurysms do not involve the coronary arteries or the valve. They are resected and continuity restored with a prosthetic graft, using the techniques already described. A more complex situation arises when the dilatation of the ascending aorta involves the aortic valve ring (annuloaortic ectasia). This situation may occur in those patients suffering from a connective tissue disorder such as Marfan's syndrome.

Surgical correction involves replacing the aortic valve and ascending aorta, and joining the coronary arteries onto the prosthesis. This is achieved by means of a 'composite graft' (Fig. 10.2) of an aortic valve prosthesis sewn into one end of a prosthetic aortic graft. The assembled graft is inserted onto the patient's valve ring proximally and onto the aorta just upstream of the innominate artery. The coronary ostia are then joined to the sides of the graft above the aortic valve.

Complications of this operation are those of any operation on the ascending aorta. Haemorrhage is the most common because of the extensive and relatively inaccessible suture lines.

False aneurysms of the ascending aorta

Most cardiac surgeons cannulate the ascending aorta for cardiopulmonary bypass, and in addition operations involving the ascending aorta – such as coronary vein graft and aortic valve replacement – are very common. False aneurysm on a suture line in the aorta is an uncommon complication but one which needs early recognition and treatment.

Pathology There has usually been some technical problem leading to less than perfect haemostasis at the aortic suture line. A small false aneurysm occurs and this may become infected. The aneurysm

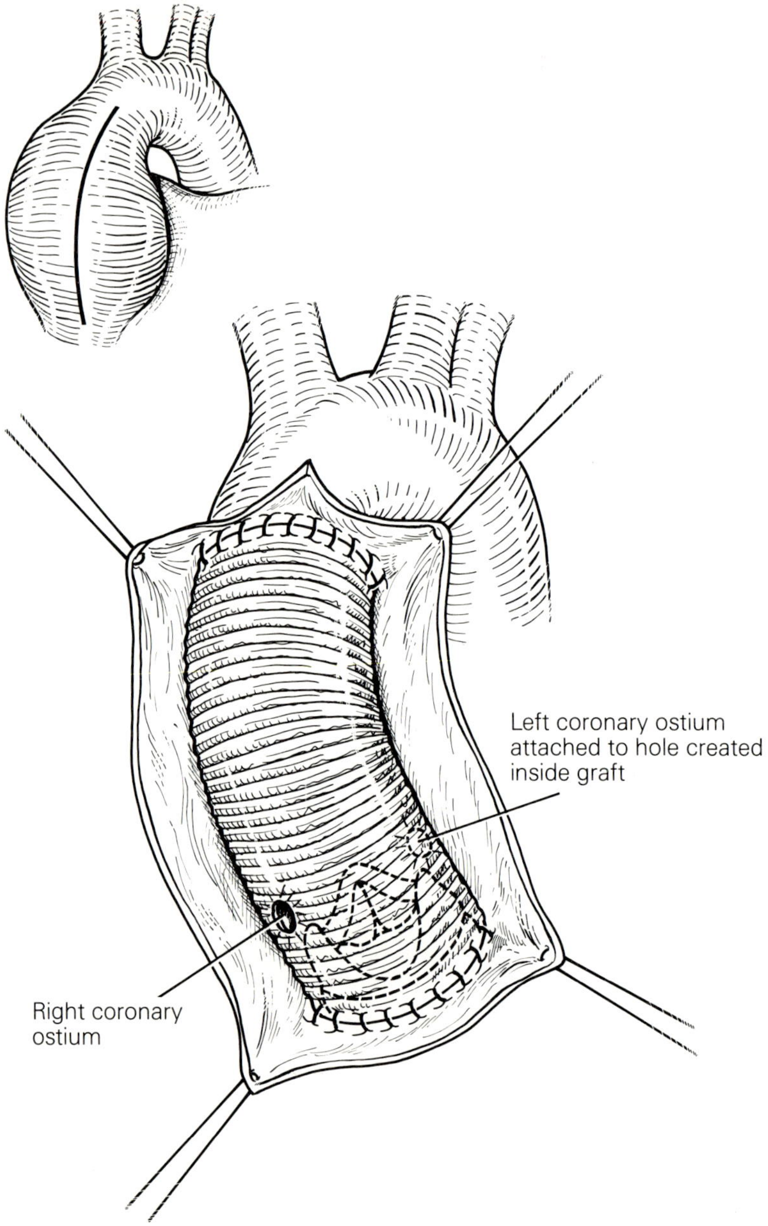

Figure 10.2 Principle of composite replacement of the ascending aorta and aortic valve.

becomes larger and larger and occupies the anterior mediastinum. The communication between the aneurysm and the aorta is usually quite small. The size of the false aneurysm may compress the heart or the superior vena cava leading to an impaired cardiac output. Eventually, the aneurysm bursts, or the patient dies of endocarditis within the lesion.

Clinical picture A patient who has had cardiac surgery presents after a few weeks with malaise and perhaps pyrexia. A chest X-ray usually shows widening of the upper mediastinum.

An aortogram will provide the diagnosis. Injection of contrast into the ascending aorta will show that there is a small leak into a large cavity anteriorly (Fig. 10.3). This leak may be very small and, unless the radiologist is aware of the pathology of the lesion, may be missed. The cavity itself rarely opacifies well.

Prevention This complication can be almost abolished by rigorous haemostasis at aortic suture lines. However, disease of the aortic wall may make this difficult to achieve and some false aneurysms do arise from this cause.

Treatment The aim of treatment is to control and close the narrow neck of the aneurysm at its origin from the ascending aorta. Once exposure has been obtained, the small size of the neck and the firm tissue of which it is composed make this easy. Usually, three or four sutures will be effective.

The major surgical problem is gaining access to the neck of the aneurysm safely without causing a fatal haemorrhage. On the six occasions the writer has performed this operation, the following procedure was developed. After anaesthesia, the patient's chest and groin are prepared. The femoral vessels are exposed and cannulated. Femorofemoral bypass is then started with cooling. When the patient's temperature reaches 30 °C, the median skin incision is reopened. When the temperature is 28 °C the circulation may be arrested safely for ten minutes. The pump flow is

Figure 10.3
Aortogram (lateral view of ascending aorta) showing contrast medium breaking into a large anterior aneurysm.

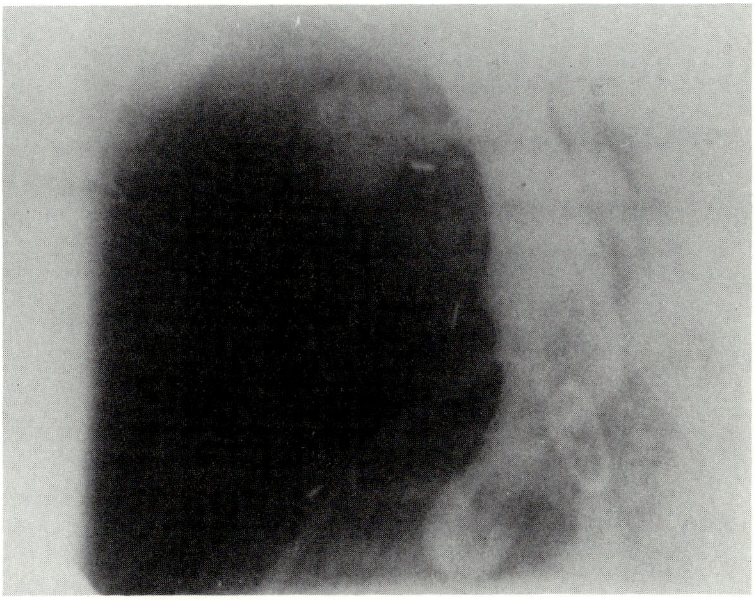

reduced to around 250–500 ml/min and the sternum rapidly opened with an electric saw. In opening the sternum, the aneurysm will be entered. The blood is sucked away and the neck of the aneurysm identified and controlled with the finger. The pump flow is then increased to the level appropriate for that temperature. Using intermittent circulatory arrest, horizontal buttressed sutures are passed through the neck of the aneurysm and control obtained.

In this experience of six patients, two have died. The first died of haemorrhage during an exploration via a right thoracotomy using femorofemoral bypass. Another died of brain damage caused by arresting the circulation for too long at 35 °C. The other four patients have left hospital without complications and, to date, no aneurysms have recurred.

Specific Problems of Operations on the Arch of the Aorta

Most operations on the arch of the aorta involve resection of an aneurysm and its replacement by a prosthetic graft. The complications are those of haemorrhage and cerebral damage. The technical problems of arch replacement are daunting. The need to join the cerebral vessels to the arch and the inaccessibility of the distal anastomosis to the descending aorta make haemorrhage very common. The practice of deep-hypothermia circulatory arrest makes effective suturing easier, as does including the anastomosis of the cerebral vessels in one suture line. Air embolism remains a major hazard.

Traumatic avulsion of a major branch of the arch

This injury may occur in any violent chest injury involving deceleration. Usually, avulsion of the innominate artery from the arch occurs, but the left carotid or the left subclavian may be affected. The avulsion involves the intima and media, the adventitia remaining intact for a while. The flow of blood into the branch may be impaired by flap occlusion of the lumen at the site of the avulsion. Ultimately, rupture will occur in most cases. Rarely, a false aneurysm, often calcified, will be found much later.

Diagnosis The injury should be suspected in every patient with a severe chest injury. Examination of the pulses in the upper limbs and neck may show an abnormality. The chest X-ray may show a widened upper mediastinum. A fracture of the first rib should raise the suspicion of an avulsion, not because of a direct causal relationship but because fracture of this relatively protected rib indicates severe trauma to the chest (Fig. 10.4).

The only accurate method of diagnosis is by aortography and it seems certain that this investigation is not used widely enough in

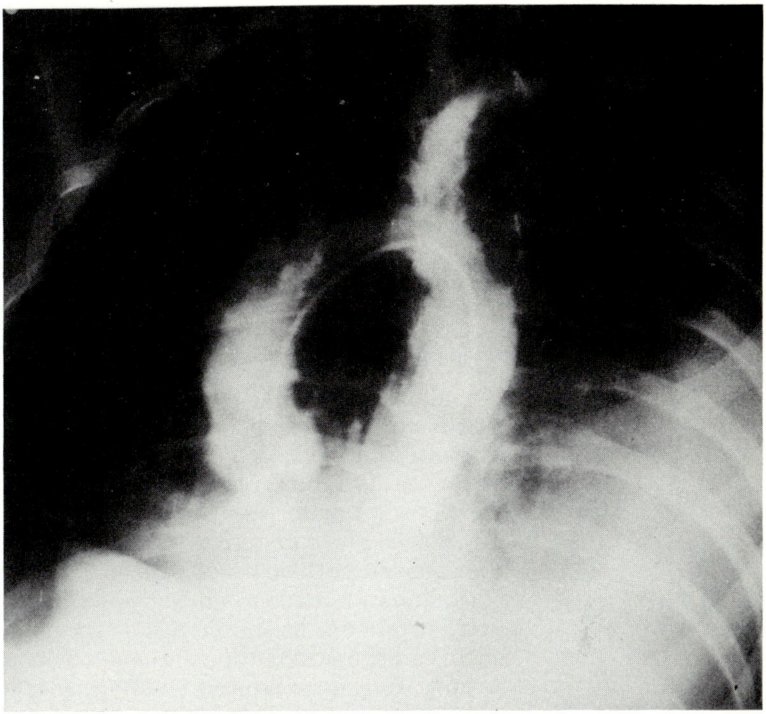

Figure 10.4
Aortogram showing descending aorta with extravasation of blood around aortic isthmus.

patients with severe chest injuries. Lacerations of the arch and descending aorta are frequently found at postmortem in patients dying from chest injury. The complexity of the clinical situation and the difficulties of clinical diagnosis, coupled with the near certainty of a fatal outcome of aortic lacerations, should lead to aortography being much more frequently performed. If some negative investigations result, it is a price worth paying if fewer patients die unnecessarily from these highly treatable problems.

Surgical repair is performed under cardiopulmonary bypass and side-clamping of the aorta and the avulsed vessel. The operating surgeon should not be dismayed when he first exposes the site of the injury. The external appearances of the lesion may be disappointing – merely a 'haematoma'. Only when the 'haematoma' is excised does the extent of the avulsion become apparent.

Specific Problems of Operations on the Descending Aorta

Dissection

Dissection of the aorta may begin as a tear in the intima and media just below the origin of the left subclavian artery. The principles of surgical correction remain the same as those described for correction of dissections of the ascending aorta, but the timing of surgery differs. In most descending or 'posterior' dissections, the danger of bursting and haemorrhage is low, provided the blood pressure can be kept down to a low normal level. Urgent surgery is only performed if there seems to be compromise of a major branch of the aorta or if rupture occurs.

Coarctation

This lesion and its complications are discussed in Chapter 9.

Aneurysm

There are no specific complications, other than those already described both for aneurysm and operations on the descending aorta.

Traumatic transection

This is a more common lesion than avulsion of the major branches of the arch of the aorta. Typically, the tear occurs in the descending aorta, just below the origin of the left subclavian artery (see Fig. 4.3). The pathology and outcome of the lesion are the same as in the case of avulsion from the arch.

Diagnosis is made by aortography. A wide mediastinum should raise suspicions as should a rightward deviation of the endotracheal or nasogastric tube in the unconscious, ventilated patient. Aortography must be more widely used if patients are not to die of this correctable lesion.

Urgent operation is advised. Visceral protection with left atriofemoral or femorofemoral bypass, or the use of the heparinized shunt, is used by most surgeons. The affected aorta may be directly repaired or replaced with a prosthetic graft. The complications of treatment are those of any operation on the descending aorta.

Summary

Operations on the thoracic aorta usually involve the insertion of a prosthesis and infection of this prosthesis is a fatal combination. Haemorrhage is common and is largely avoidable by an appropriate surgical technique sealing off the graft and by the use of fresh blood.

Visceral damage is common after operations on the thoracic aorta and depending on the area being operated on, measures to protect specific organs must be used. Most visceral damage can be prevented, but spinal cord injury is a danger which cannot be entirely predicted or prevented.

Persisting controversies

- The liberal use of aortography in the early diagnosis of trauma to the thoracic aorta.

- The most suitable method of affording visceral protection, particularly of the brain and spinal cord.
- The place of the intraluminal graft in the surgery of aortic dissection.
- The safest way to manage false aneurysms of the ascending aorta.

Conclusion

The thoracic aorta remains one of the most daunting challenges facing the surgeon and in no other part of surgery will technical imperfections be so ruthlessly and rapidly exposed. Visceral protection is necessary in every case. Infection of an aortic prosthesis will usually be fatal. Nevertheless, with experience and careful planning of surgery, many of these complications can be avoided and in this area above all others the avoidance of complications, rather than their treatment, must be given preference.

Further reading

Anagnostopoulos, C.E. (1975) *Acute Aortic Dissections.* Baltimore: University Park Press.

Krause, A.H., Ferguson, T.B. & Weldon, C.S. (1972) Thoracic aneurysmectomy using the Idmac heparin shunt. *Ann. Thorac. Surg.*, *14*, 123.

Ross, D.N., Frazier, T.G. & Gonzalez Lavin, L. (1972) Surgery of Marfan's syndrome and related conditions of the aortic root (annulo-aortic ectasia). *Thorax*, *27*, 52.

Symbas, P.N., Tyras, D.H., Ware, R.E. & Dioro, P.A. (1973) Traumatic rupture of the aorta. *Ann. Surg.*, *178*, 6.

Valiathan, M.S., Weldon, C.S., Bender, H.W., Topaz, S.R. & Gott, V.L. (1968) Resection of aneurysms of the descending aorta using a GBH-coated shunt bypass. *J. Surg. Res.*, *8*, 197.

11 Drug-related Complications in Cardiopulmonary Surgery

Most patients needing cardiopulmonary operations are already taking a number of drugs. These drugs are both powerful and dangerous. They have specific side-effects and, in addition, the surgical operation often exposes an additional set of problems. Even if no additional problems arise, there is the need to decide whether or not a drug should be continued over the operative period and, if so, by what route and in what dosage it should be administered. In this chapter, the complications of drug treatment affecting the lungs and cardiac surgery will be outlined separately.

Lung Surgery (Table 11.1)

Corticosteroids

These drugs are frequently taken by patients who are referred with chronic inflammatory lung disease, such as fibrosing alveolitis. These patients are referred for open-lung biopsy or removal of a solitary lesion. Some patients will be taking steroids for diseases situated outside the thorax.

The general side-effects of steroids will affect the surgery. Suppression of the pituitary drive to the adrenal cortex will cause metabolic problems in the postoperative period unless the dosage of steroids is increased during this time. It is usual to give an increased dose of corticosteroid – usually hydrocortisone 100 mg i.v. every six hours – beginning with the premedication and continuing for three days. After that, the dosage may be reduced to the normal for that patient over another three or four days. Such a regimen is immunosuppressive to a degree and the possibility of infection becoming established must be considered. Especially scrupulous attention to aseptic technique in the operating theatre and the intensive care ward is needed. Should infection occur, the normal clinical manifestation may be attenuated by the drugs.

Long-term steroid therapy causes technical problems for the

Table 11.1
Drugs given to patients undergoing lung surgery.

Drug	Indication
1 Corticosteroids	Anti-inflammatory action
	Suppression of allergic bronchospasm
2 Bronchodilators	Bronchospasm
3 Antibiotics	Chronic lung disease

surgeon. All the tissues become more fragile and the surgical technique must accommodate to this fact. The chest wall should be opened with meticulous haemostasis and closed equally carefully. Often pericostal sutures may be needed in order to close the chest securely. Blood vessel walls are also weakened by the drug and the larger vessels should be controlled by a suture technique rather than relying on ligatures. Smaller vessels should be controlled by ligature rather than diathermy.

Bronchodilators
Patients with chronic obstructive airways disease can develop surgical disease of the lungs. Most such patients are taking a bronchodilator, usually a β-adrenoceptor stimulant, such as salbutamol. Without the drug, such patients rapidly develop airways obstruction. The drug is usually consumed up to the time of the operation. During the operation and postoperative period, the bronchodilating action of salbutamol may be achieved by its inhalation and there are devices available which attach to either the oxygen mask or ventilators and effectively nebulize the drug into the inspired air. Salbutamol should be used with caution in patients with ischaemic heart disease.

In an emergency, where severe bronchospasm suddenly occurs, intravenous aminophylline (250 mg for an adult) will provide effective bronchodilation. Adrenaline, although an effective bronchodilator, has many undesirable side-effects and should not be used. If aminophylline is used, it must be given over a period of at least ten minutes. The use of aminophylline as an emergency, however, is a reflection of inadequate bronchodilation therapy and the use of nebulized salbutamol will avoid many sudden crises.

Antibiotics
Some patients with chronic lung disease, such as bronchiectasis and chronic bronchitis, have been taking broad spectrum antibiotics for months or years before they see the surgeon. The reason for referrral to the surgeon may be related to the need to take antibiotics, such as the need for resection of bronchiectasis or an infected lung cyst. The surgical lung condition may be a separate issue, such as bronchial carcinoma developing in a patient with chronic bronchitis.

Long-term antibiotic therapy alters the bacterial flora of the patient. The resistance to overgrowth with resistant organisms is lower, and frequently these patients have a variety of resistant and often bizarre organisms in their sputum. The surgeon is concerned that these organisms, tolerated in the medical patient, may cause pulmonary infection or septicaemia after a lung operation.

If the antibiotics can be stopped for a period of several weeks before the operation, the organisms found may revert back to the usual contaminants of the sputum found in normal individuals. During this time, the patient should be treated by frequent physiotherapy and postural drainage. The operation may then proceed with the usual antibiotic prophylaxis favoured by the surgeon. Often, however, either the patient cannot tolerate any withdrawal of antibiotics or the sputum remains contaminated with resistant organisms. The wrong response to this dilemma is to search for and administer some exotic and specific antibiotic since this will merely alter the pattern of resistance and sensitivity of the organisms contaminating the sputum. The correct response is to perform surgery forthwith, accepting that if infection occurs it is going to be difficult to treat effectively. When infection does occur, the specific antibiotic is given together with physiotherapy. The difference lies in the antibiotic treatment of bacterial contamination as opposed to bacterial infection.

Summary

Patients with surgical lung lesions are often taking a variety of drugs. Steroids, bronchodilators and antibiotics all pose problems for the surgeon. Steroid regimens will need augmentation around the time of the operation and infection is a danger. Bronchodilators may be given by nebulizer throughout the operative period and in an emergency intravenous aminophylline may be needed.

Long-term antibiotic treatment alters the bacterial flora of the whole patient and in particular the contaminants of the sputum. Ideally, antibiotics should be stopped for several weeks before operation, but if this is not possible the surgeon may have to operate against a background of exotic bacterial contamination. Only if *infection* occurs should antibiotics be given.

Cardiac Surgery

Most adult and some paediatric cardiac surgical patients are taking drugs before operation (Table 11.2). The surgeon needs to review the indications and necessity for each drug before surgery. Some drugs will be needed, especially those preventing or reducing cardiac failure or ischaemia, and if these are stopped the patient will be harmed. Thus, although a drug such as

Table 11.2
Drugs given to patients undergoing cardiac surgery.

1 Drugs acting on the myocardium:
 (a) Cardiac glycosides (digoxin)
 (b) β-Adrenergic blockers
 (c) Calcium antagonists
2 Drugs acting on the vessels (vasodilators):
 (a) Sodium nitroprusside
 (b) Nitrates
 (c) Calcium antagonists
3 Diuretics and potassium supplements
4 Drugs acting on the clotting mechanism:
 (a) Heparin
 (b) Protamine

frusemide should ideally be stopped before operation, it is undesirable to have a patient who develops pulmonary oedema at the time of arrival in the operating theatre. There can be no general rules; each patient has a specific and unique problem needing consideration.

Drugs acting on the myocardium

Digoxin This is a commonly given drug, usually in a dosage of 250 μg/day for the adult patient. Although digoxin has an inotropic action, its main indication for use is the presence of atrial fibrillation. If atrial fibrillation is not present, many surgeons discontinue the drug before surgery, recognizing that it takes several days before the myocardium is free of the drug.

Atrial fibrillation before surgery should lead to the drug being given up to the time of the operation. During the operation, digoxin in small intravenous doses (125 μg) may be needed to control rapid ventricular rates in atrial fibrillation. After the operation, it is usual to give 125 μg of digoxin intravenously every six hours until the patient can resume oral medication. Extra doses are needed if there is uncontrolled atrial fibrillation. If facilities for the estimation of serum digoxin levels are available, they should be used provided it is understood that a meaningful answer is only given if the serum is taken at least five hours after the last intravenous dose. If a fully digitalized patient (serum digoxin 2 ng/ml) has a persistently uncontrolled ventricular rate due to atrial fibrillation, the use of a cardioselective β-blocker such as acebutolol (5 mg) will help to slow the rate.

The clinical effect of digoxin toxicity may be blunted by surgery. Nausea and vomiting may be due to other causes and true bigeminal rhythm with alternate beats being due to ventricular extrasystoles is not common. Conversely a low serum potassium level will make worse a tendency to digoxin toxicity.

There is no universal agreement among surgeons about the indications and use for digoxin. There are those who prefer to use digoxin only in atrial fibrillation but others use it on all cases of acquired heart disease, whether in atrial fibrillation or not. This division of opinion reflects the differing opinions about the indications for digoxin therapy in the medical community at large. While there is much logic in restricting the use of digoxin to patients with atrial fibrillation, it cannot be denied that the drug is useful in patients with congestive heart failure and sinus rhythm. The side-effects of digoxin appear at serum levels not greatly exceeding a normal therapeutic level and it is for this reason that many physicians prefer its restricted use.

Summary. Digoxin is given to patients in atrial fibrillation throughout the perioperative period, with the aim of controlling the ventricular rate. The margin between therapeutic and toxic levels is small and therefore digoxin is infrequently used for its known inotropic effect.

Persisting controversy

- The indications for the wider use of digoxin at the time of cardiac surgery.

β-Adrenergic blockers

These drugs reduce the force of contraction of the myocardium and therefore reduce its oxygen demand. In ischaemia, therefore, these drugs reduce symptoms of angina and certainly help to prevent a subsequent infarction in those patients who have had a previous infarct; they may also help those patients who have not yet had an infarct.

β-Blockers are available in many types, each with a different duration and selectivity of action. It is unlikely that any one individual can remember and be familiar with all the available types and it is desirable that the surgeon and cardiologist should become thoroughly familiar with the use of one or two only. β-Blockers vary in their length of action and in their degree of selectivity. Some act mainly on the myocardium and others affect β-adrenergic activity thoughout the body. For instance, propranolol, which is a widely used β-blocker, is relatively unselective. As well as slowing and reducing the force of the heart beat, it may cause bronchospasm and provoke or aggravate peripheral limb ischaemia. Many patients taking propranolol complain of nightmares and lassitude.

Nearly all patients who need a coronary bypass operation are taking β-blocking drugs. It is known that the abrupt cessation of such medication may possibly cause a myocardial infarction. The commonest practice is to continue β-blockers up to the time of surgery, so that there may be maximum protection for the myocardium in the crucial period between induction of anaesthesia and the beginning of cardiopulmonary bypass.

Nonselective β-blockers may cause complications during and after bypass. The peripheral tissue utilization and handling of potassium seems to be impaired, particularly by propranolol. The result is a high level of serum potassium and this can interfere with the force of contraction of the heart after bypass. Only when the serum potassium has been lowered will the heart resume effective action. Awareness of this problem will lead to the patient being given little or no potassium supplements during the operation.

After the operation, β-blockers are stopped in most cases, but if a smaller but continuing dose of the same drug is given over the first few postoperative weeks, there seems to be a smaller incidence of disabling arrhythmia.

Summary. β-Adrenergic blocking drugs are extremely powerful and are widely used in the symptomatic treatment of ischaemic heart disease. There are many different types of β-blocker, each with its own specific plasma half-life and degree of cardioselectivity. β-Blockers are usually continued up to the time of operation in order to prevent critical ischaemia occurring. Hyperkalaemia is a hazard of β-blockade which can depress cardiac action.

Persisting controversies

- The use of low dose β-blocker after coronary artery operations.
- The best β-blocker for surgical patients.

Calcium antagonists

This group of drugs (e.g. nifedipine, verapamil) blocks the uptake of calcium within vessel walls and within the myocardium. Partly as a result of vasodilatation and partly as a result of the diminished force of cardiac systole, the myocardial oxygen demands are reduced and ischaemia lessened. The drugs, particularly nifedipine, are widely used in the medical treatment of ischaemic heart disease. The body of experience suggests that the drugs may be safely continued up to the time of surgery. However, several surgeons have encountered sudden and otherwise unexplained postoperative cardiac arrests in such patients. These reports, being anecdotal, need treating with extreme caution and they have certainly not influenced the majority of cardiac surgeons in their policies.

Summary. Calcium antagonists are widely used in the treatment of ischaemic heart disease and do not appear to pose any specific problems at the time of surgery. However, caution in giving such powerful drugs in the perioperative period is advised. Nifedipine has no antiarrhythmic activity.

Drugs acting on the blood vessels

This group of drugs causes vasodilatation, and are widely used by the oral route in the medical treatment of ischaemic heart disease. Vasodilatation reduces the peripheral resistance and thus lowers cardiac work whilst allowing an increase in cardiac output. This action is valuable under two circumstances: first, the ischaemic myocardium must be helped by any reduction in work and therefore oxygen demand; and second, the failing heart with a low cardiac output will be considerably helped by vasodilatation of the peripheral vascular system, which leads to a reduction of cardiac work and an elevation of the cardiac output.

Vasodilators in cardiac failure after operation

The need at this time and with such an unstable situation is for a vasodilator which is quickly effective and with a very short duration of action. Intravenous sodium nitroprusside acts mainly on arterioles and intravenous nitroglycerin preparations act on both arterioles and venules. Nitroprusside therefore reduces the afterload of the heart of the emptying pressure, whereas nitroglycerin preparations reduce both the afterload and the filling pressures of the heart (preload). Of the two, more experience has been gained in the use of sodium nitroprusside, but this drug has tissue toxicity side-effects which may emerge at doses of more than 8 $\mu g/kg \cdot min^{-1}$. These show themselves as metabolic acidosis due to tissue hypoxia. Nitroglycerin does not have these side-effects.

Both drugs are administered intravenously by an electronically controlled infusion. The patient must have full cardiac monitoring in order to detect if these drugs are having the desired effect. Measurements of right and left atrial pressure, arterial pressure and preferably of cardiac output should be made repeatedly. In most patients, there will be a rise in cardiac output which is reflected in an increased tissue perfusion. However, the arterial pressure may be unduly affected and lead to the drugs being curtailed before the desired increase in cardiac output is achieved.

Both drugs are only suitable for use in the intensive care ward, and they must never be used unless the patient is fully monitored. Long acting vasodilators such as chlorpromazine suffer from side-effects and by the fact that once given, their action is not readily reversed if appropriate.

A new oral vasodilator which works by inhibiting the formation and action of angiotensin II has now been made available for clinical use (Captopril). This appears to be effective in the long-term management of left ventricular failure.

Summary. Vasodilators lead to decreased cardiac work and an increased cardiac output. Vasodilator therapy of low output syndrome is now well established and effective, provided that full cardiac monitoring is available. Short acting intravenous vasodilators are used so that inappropriate responses can be terminated abruptly.

Persisting controversy

- Is nitroprusside in any way superior to nitroglycerin?

Vasodilators in the treatment of ischaemic heart disease

These drugs are of two types: the calcium antagonists and the nitrate preparations. Both are given orally. They pose no special problems to the surgeon except that they cause skin vasodilatation and this may make incisions bleed very freely. Haematomas may occur in the legs where the saphenous vein is harvested. Patients frequently complain of headaches with the use of these drugs.

Diuretics and potassium supplements

Diuretics are given to many patients with heart disease and reduce the amount of pulmonary congestion and oedema. They are usually needed up to the time of the operation. Although there are many types of diuretic in clinical use at this time, frusemide or its derivatives are the most widely used. It acts on the ascending loop of Henle in the renal tubule, is associated with a predictable response and is virtually free of toxicity. It may be given intravenously or orally.

The surgeon faces especial difficulties with frusemide particularly, but also with other diuretics. The increase in urinary output is associated with an unpredictable and perhaps severe loss of potassium in the urine and a low serum potassium will produce a serious arrhythmia, especially if the patient is digitalized. Since the serum potassium is only a small part of the total body potassium, there is no detectable difference in the total body potassium as a result of diuretic therapy. However, it is clinical practice to add potassium supplements to the drug regimen of a patient receiving a diuretic. A patient on the intensive care ward will have regular and frequent estimations made of the serum potassium and appropriate adjustments made.

The patient receiving oral diuretics will usually take a potassium preparation as well (usually Slow-K – a sustained release preparation). This may cause nausea and vomiting. Certain patients are at risk from small bowel ulceration and in those patients with any oesophageal hold-up (as in those with a dilated left atrium) the tablets may cause chemical erosion of the oesophageal mucosa.

Liquid potassium supplements are available and there are many proprietary types of potassium tablet. No patient on long-term diuretic treatment should be denied potassium supplements – the choice of a particular type which suits the patient may be more difficult.

Drugs acting on the clotting mechanism

Anticoagulation is widely used in cardiothoracic surgery for the following:

1 Prophylaxis against venous thromboembolism.
2 During cardiopulmonary bypass.
3 Long-term anticoagulation after prosthetic valve replacement.

Prophylaxis against venous thromboembolism

Ample evidence exists that the perioperative use of low-dose subcutaneous heparin calcium helps to prevent venous thromboembolism in patients having major surgery. Most cardiothoracic surgeons favour its use in all patients, apart from those having procedures involving cardiopulmonary bypass. No special hazards are encountered by the surgeon and there does not seem to be an increase in the amount of blood lost during the operation.

During cardiopulmonary bypass

As stated previously, heparin is given before cannulation and bypass. It is reversed with protamine when the cannulas are removed. The major complication associated with the use of heparin is that, for some reason, it may not be given to the patient. Each surgeon should make sure that the system for giving heparin is foolproof. If he cannot be sure that a reliable anaesthetic colleague will give the drug into a properly placed venous catheter, the surgeon is obliged to draw up the drug and inject it directly into the circulation with the chest open. Failure to give heparin properly will lead to thrombosis within the heart–lung circuit and a total inability of blood clotting in the patient, usually resulting in death.

At the end of cardiopulmonary bypass, the action of heparin is reversed by the use of protamine. This drug is a biological product. Its injection is associated with peripheral vasodilatation and some depression of cardiac action, and it is usually given very slowly into a peripheral vein over a period of 20 minutes. Some evidence has been produced to show that direct injection into the aorta will avoid some of these problems or at least alleviate them. The mechanism of this is unknown, but is probably related to the effects of protamine on the pulmonary circulation. On occasions, the administration of protamine will lead to pulmonary oedema and a low left atrial pressure. This may be an allergic reaction to a biological product. It is treated by restarting bypass and the administration of corticosteroids.

Long-term anticoagulation after prosthetic valve replacement

Anticoagulants are used after most valve replacements. In mechanical valve replacement, anticoagulants are usually continued for life. In biological valve replacements, the need for anticoagulants is less, and if a patient is in sinus rhythm, it is often possible to stop anticoagulants three months after operation.

There are no special surgical complications of the use of oral anticoagulants after valve replacement. Three features do need attention, however:

1. The effective starting dose for oral anticoagulation is lower after cardiopulmonary bypass. Warfarin at 4 mg will achieve the effect of 10 mg in other patients.
2. Anticoagulants should not be started too soon after valve replacement because of the fear of haemopericardium and tamponade. In practice, to begin oral anticoagulants at four days after surgery is safe.

3 The patient on anticoagulants who presents for a surgical operation – often of an emergency nature – causes particular worry. If the procedure is one not involving cardiopulmonary bypass, such as a lung or abdominal operation, the operation may be safely performed without stopping the anticoagulants, as long as that the clotting ratio (BCR) remains at about twice normal. The worst possible action is to stop anticoagulants in a patient with a prosthetic valve replacement. Even major abdominal surgery can be performed without a noticeable increase in blood loss under the normal range of anticoagulation which is safe for a patient with a prosthetic cardiac valve.

If the patient needs an emergency cardiac operation, the effects of oral anticoagulants may be reversed by giving fresh frozen plasma after the bypass has been finished. The routine cardiac reoperation should be preceded by stopping oral anticoagulants three days before surgery. Any prolongation of the clotting ratio on the morning of surgery should be treated by the injection of vitamin K.

Summary Oral anticoagulants are used in cardiothoracic surgery to prevent venous thromboembolism, during cardiopulmonary bypass and to prevent thromboembolism from prosthetic valves. Complications arise mostly from their use in patients who have had valve replacements. Patients with mechanical prostheses should receive anticoagulants for life, but some patients with biological valves may stop them after a few months. Further surgical operations on anticoagulated patients should be done without stopping anticoagulants as this leads to a high incidence of valve thrombosis and thromboembolism.

Persisting controversy

- Does fresh blood help to reverse the effects of warfarin better than fresh frozen plasma?

Conclusions

Each drug used by cardiologists in the treatment of heart and lung disease will cause specific problems at the time of surgery. The need for such drugs, however, continues at least up to the time of operation and the surgeon must become familiar with their actions. Of the drugs affecting the myocardium, the use of digoxin remains the most controversial, many surgeons using it only in the presence of aerial fibrillation. β-blockers should be continued until operation in patients with ischaemic heart disease because of the dangers of a myocardial infarction. The newer vasodilator drugs have proven effective not only in the treatment of the failing left ventricle but also in the intensive care ward in the treatment of low output syndrome. The possibility of a drug-related complication must be considered in every patient undergoing cardiothoracic surgery.

12 Surgery and Disorders of Cardiac Rhythm and Pacing

A common complication of any type of cardiothoracic operation is the onset of an abnormal cardiac rhythm. In most hospital patients, arrhythmias are the concern of the general physician or cardiologist. In cardiothoracic surgical patients, however, the surgeon must manage the problem because of the urgency of the situation and because some of the causes are surgical in origin. Hence the cardiothoracic surgeon needs to acquire a knowledge of these conditions which surgeons in other specialties can leave to others.

The normal rhythm of the heart is sinus, i.e. the contraction of the atria occurs before the contraction of the ventricles and the two events are co-ordinated by the conducting mechanism of the heart, namely the atrioventricular (AV) node and the bundle of His. The contraction of the atria drives blood through the atrioventricular valves and stretches the ventricular myocardium. The subsequent ventricular contraction is therefore much stronger because of Starling's law of the heart. Once any other rhythm than sinus occurs, a significant fall in ventricular performance and hence cardiac output will occur. Since many cardiothoracic patients have a compromised cardiac output at best, any further fall can be enough to be quickly damaging. A second reason for concern with arrhythmias is the unstable nature of some types. Many arrhythmias untreated will progress to cardiac arrest and in cardiothoracic patients, in particular, this may happen very quickly.

A surgical approach to cardiac arrhythmias is therefore germane to the training of a cardiothoracic surgeon. To the physician specializing in these conditions, the surgical approach will seem naïve and simplistic. Nevertheless, most arrhythmias will in practice be dealt with by surgeons and only the less common or resistant problems will present themselves to the specialist physician.

Definitions. The acceptable cardiac rhythm after surgery is sinus at a rate of between 79 and 100 beats per minute. Any other rhythm or rate is potentially damaging and, for the purposes of this chapter, termed an arrhythmia (Table 12.1).

Table 12.1
Cardiac arrhythmias.

1 Complete heart block
2 Disorders of rate (but basic rhythm sinus)
   (a) Tachycardia
   (b) Bradycardia
3 Disorders of rhythm (and perhaps of rate)

Diagnosis of Arrhythmia

Most patients with a cardiac arrhythmia are attached to an oscilloscope monitor of the electrocardiograph. This device is inadequate for the purpose of diagnosing the nature of this disorder. Ideally, a full 12-lead electrocardiograph tracing should be made, but if circumstances do not permit this a tracing of the rhythm on a single strip will suffice. Only by the careful analysis of a paper tracing can a precise diagnosis be made.

Complete Heart Block

This disorder may occur after any form of cardiac surgery if myocardial protection has been inadequate. Some operations, such as repair of a ventricular septal defect or aortic valve replacement, are conducted very close to the AV node and bundle of His and there may be surgical damage causing AV dissociation and consequent slow idioventricular rhythm. Usually, the onset of complete AV block causes a very inadequate cardiac output and even asystole may follow. Early recognition and treatment are therefore essential.

Recognition
The electrocardiogram (ECG) will show wide idioventricular complexes occurring at a much slower rate (30–50/min in adults) than the P waves due to atrial contraction.

Treatment
Any patient having cardiac surgery runs the risk of developing AV block and perhaps asystole. All patients at risk, and to many surgeons that means *every* patient, should have a temporary epicardial ventricular pacing wire inserted during the operation. The large majority of these will never be used and will be removed by traction just before the patient leaves hospital. In those cases where AV block does occur, however, the ability to start electrical pacing quickly may be life saving. Other treatments are inferior and lack the rapidity and control of electrical pacing. In an emergency the idioventricular rate may be increased by a chronotropic drug such as isoprenaline given as a constant intravenous infusion (4 mg in 500 ml isotonic saline at about 20 ml/h). The potential for asystole to occur remains, however,

and persistent AV block must be managed electrically. If no epicardial lead is present, one must be passed by the intravenous route into the right ventricle.

Sinus Tachycardia

Sinus tachycardia is defined as sinus rhythm at a rate of more than 110/min in the adult and more than 150/min in children. The cardiac output is usually good. The concern is that the period of coronary filling in diastole may be so reduced as to impair myocardial oxygen supply.

There are four major causes of sinus tachycardia which are of concern to the surgeon. These are:

1 Hypovolaemia.
2 Hypoxia.
3 Cardiac tamponade.
4 Pain and apprehension.

Each of these causes has implications for the patient's survival and the tachycardia is not the primary disorder but more a reflection of it.

Hypovolaemia may be excluded by measurement of the ventricular filling pressures. Hypoxia may be detected by measurement of the arterial blood gases. In each case, the cause of the primary problem should be discovered and treated appropriately.

Pain and apprehension release catecholamines which cause tachycardia, but so do hypoxia and hypovolaemia. If tachycardia persists after relief of pain, the possibility of cardiac tamponade must be considered. The surgical disorder or the operation which a patient has had may not lead to cardiac tamponade, of course, but if the tachycardia follows a cardiac operation this diagnosis must be carefully considered. Ultimately, the only way to prove the question conclusively will be to reopen the chest.

Treatment

The treatment lies in the accurate diagnosis and removal of the underlying cause. However, in some patients, a sinus tachycardia will persist in the absence of any discernible cause and this situation is found usually after a coronary artery operation, possibly as a result of withdrawal of adrenergic blocking drugs. The attending surgeon then has to consider the quality of the operation (was successful and total revascularization achieved?) and decide whether to accept the situation or to try a small dose of β-blocking drugs. This decision can only be made, however, when the more serious causes have been excluded.

Summary

Sinus tachycardia may not cause low cardiac output, but may prejudice myocardial oxygen delivery. Hypoxia, hypovolaemia and cardiac tamponade have to be excluded before assuming that the tachycardia is a result of pain and apprehension. Once these causes are excluded, the surgeon has to decide whether to accept the situation or to treat it with small doses of β-blockers.

Persisting controversy

- The use of digoxin in patients with sinus rhythm.

Sinus Bradycardia

A heart rate of below 70 beats per minute may occur after cardiac surgery and is usually related to the preoperative use of β-blocking drugs in ischaemic heart disease. The cardiac output is usually good and, if the rhythm is stable, the situation is acceptable, particularly with reference to coronary filling. Frequently, however, the idioventricular rhythm breaks through and gives rise to ventricular extrasystoles. These appear as wide, slurred QRS complexes on the ECG (Fig. 12.1). In these circumstances, the heart rate should be increased. There are two ways of accomplishing this: first, by atrial pacing and second, by the use of chronotropic drugs such as isoprenaline. Those surgeons who routinely place atrial and ventricular pacing wires at the time of surgery will use pacing. Others will need to use isoprenaline as an infusion. Ventricular pacing alone is the least efficient of all since the normal atrial contraction or 'kick' to the ventricles is lost.

Very often, sinus bradycardia will resolve when the patient breathes spontaneously after surgery. Less common causes of a sinus bradycardia are cerebral swelling, due to oedema or to carbon dioxide retention, and jaundice. In each of these cases, however, the bradycardia is clearly a secondary problem.

A final point must be made in this section on the management of disorders of sinus rhythm. Physicians tend to get very excited about 'first degree heart block'. This condition exists when the interval between the P wave of the ECG and the onset of the QRS complex exceeds 220 msec, but the normal 1:1 relationship is preserved. From the surgical viewpoint, first degree heart block is irrelevant (Fig. 12.2).

Summary

Sinus bradycardia (including first degree heart block) is a benign condition unless low cardiac output or ventricular extrasystoles occur. Electrical pacing of the atria or the infusion of isoprenaline will increase the rate to acceptable levels. Ventricular pacing, although increasing the rate, will often reduce cardiac output by creating an uncoordinated pattern of ventricular contraction.

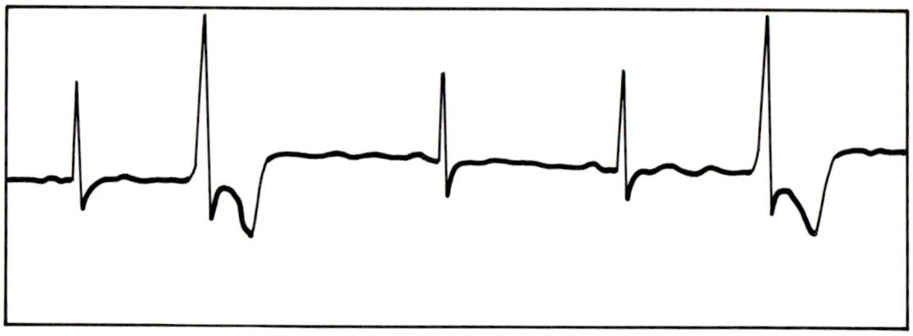

Figure 12.1
ECG showing a bradycardia with 'breakthrough' ventricular extrasystoles.

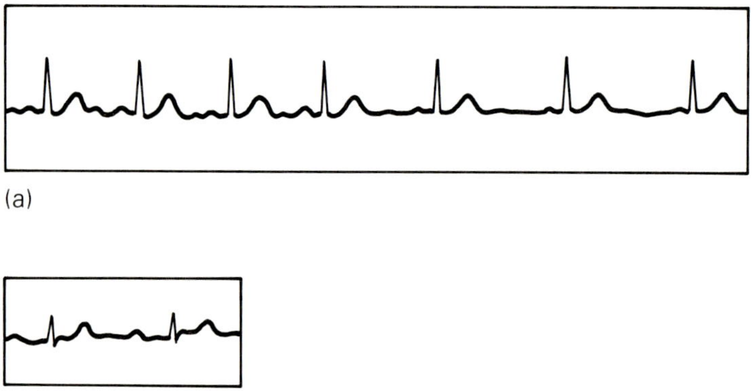

(a) (b)

Figure 12.2
(a) ECG with normal sinus rhythm (PR interval less than 200 msec). (b) ECG showing first degree heart block (PR interval greater than 200 msec).

Disorders of Cardiac Rhythm

In general, all of these disorders reduce cardiac output and usually need urgent treatment. An expectant attitude will lead to the death of many patients.

There are two types of rhythm disorder, and the difference lies in the origin of the abnormality and the stability of the condition. Those disorders arising in the atria cause tachycardias and lower cardiac output, but usually do not cause cardiac arrest as a consequence. These are the supraventricular arrhythmias. Disorders arising in the ventricles also cause tachycardias, but are very unstable and liable to go abruptly into cardiac arrest. This distinction between supraventricular and ventricular arrhythmias is a fundamental one of causation, complications and treatment.

Supraventricular arrhythmias

Atrial fibrillation and atrial flutter

These two arrhythmias frequently occur after surgery of the heart. Their onset is sudden and the pulse rises to 160–180/min. The cardiac output falls, the skin temperature falls, the urine output drops and the arterial blood pressure is reduced. Diagnosis is made by the rhythm strip of the electrocardiograph or a full 12-lead recording (Fig. 12.3). In each, the QRS complex is unchanged (except that very rarely a rate-induced bundle branch block may occur – see below, page 227).

In atrial fibrillation, a good recording will show loss of P waves and an irregular QRS complex (Fig. 12.3a). Because of the rate, care must be taken to measure accurately the intervals between R waves because the differences between irregular complex may differ only slightly. Atrial flutter is characterized by a rate of atrial contraction of about 300–320/min. A degree of atrioventricular block exists, the ventricular rate does not rise above 180/min, and it is regular (Fig. 12.3b). In the intensive care ward, it may be impossible to obtain an ECG recording of sufficiently high quality to distinguish between the two. For practical purposes of treatment the distinction is unimportant.

Before commencing treatment, consideration needs to be given to the cause of the arrhythmia. Often, hypoxia will trigger the abnormality and disturbances of electrolytes in the serum will do likewise. Often a patient will develop a supraventricular arrhythmia if prematurely he is allowed to breathe spontaneously after surgery.

Treatment. If hypoxia is present, it should be treated. Similarly, electrolyte abnormalities (particularly of potassium) need correcting. In most patients, however, no cause for the supraventricular arrhythmias is found. In these cases, two options of treatment are available. The first is to increase the degree of atrioventricular dissociation and thus allow the ventricular rate to fall and produce a pulse rate of around 90–100/min. The second option is to restore to the atrium normal contraction and hence sinus rhythm by synchronized defibrillation. Of the two, the last is preferable because it restores the atrial 'kick' to the ventricle and provides a higher cardiac output.

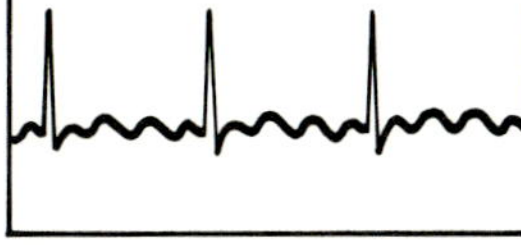

(a)

(b)

Figure 12.3 (a) ECG showing atrial fibrillation (no P waves and irregular normal QRS complexes). (b) ECG showing atrial flutter (rate 240/min with 2:1 AV block and a ventricular rate of 120/min).

The first option is to digitalize the patient. This has to be done rapidly by the intravenous route. A guide to the correct dosage lies in the patient's surface area, a measurement always known in the cardiac patient. Digitalization needs 0.6 mg/m^2 of body surface area. Half of this dose is given immediately by the intravenous route; a further one-sixth of the dose is given two hours later and four hours after that the final dose of one-sixth of the calculated digitalizing dose is given eight hours after the original injection. Digitalization by this method is safe and quickly effective. If the tachycardia persists, acebutolol in 5 mg doses intravenously up to 20 mg is used. Very few arrhythmias fail to respond to this combination.

The second option is synchronized DC defibrillation. The defibrillating shock is applied externally and starts at 100 joules. In theory, DC defibrillation should not be used on a patient who has received digoxin but in practice this makes no difference. The patient is lightly sedated for this procedure.

Atrial extrasystoles

This abnormality interrupts normal sinus rhythm by the premature interposing of an extra complex (Fig. 12.4). It has no significance and does not affect cardiac output.

Nodal rhythm

The atrioventricular node becomes the pacemaker to the heart. Conduction to the ventricles occurs normally and the atria are stimulated retrogradely. As a result, atrial and ventricular contraction are synchronous (Fig. 12.5). The abnormality is stable and only affects cardiac output by abolishing normal sinus rhythm.

Treatment may be necessary if the cardiac output drops to an unsatisfactory level. Potassium chloride (2 mmol i.v.) will often restore sinus rhythm as will speeding the heart up with intravenous isoprenaline (2 mg in 500 ml isotonic saline at 5–20 ml/h depending on the heart rate achieved).

Summary

Supraventricular arrhythmias are common after cardiac operations. Their significance lies in the consequent reduction of cardiac output and not in their inherent instability. The QRS complex is normal. Accurate diagnosis depends on the rhythm strip or 12-lead electrocardiograph, but fine distinctions between atrial fibrillation and flutter are not always possible. After excluding remediable causes such as hypoxia, the patient may be

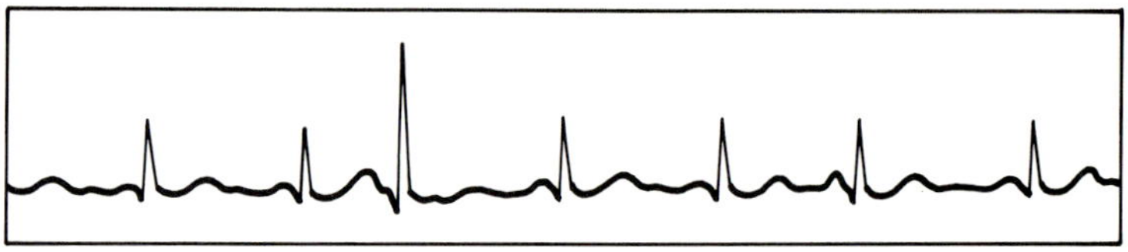

Figure 12.4 ECG showing atrial extrasystoles (irregular P waves followed by a normal QRS complex).

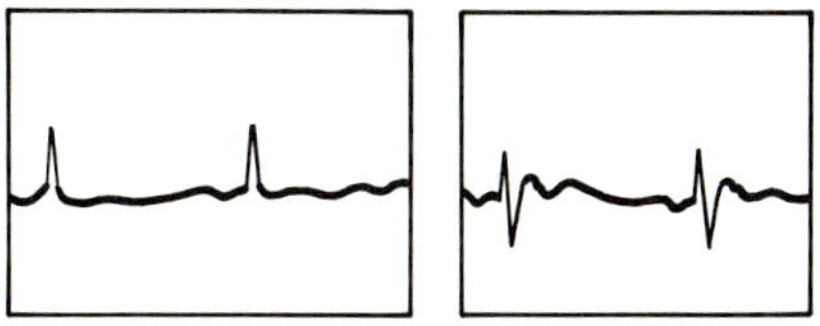

Figure 12.5
ECG showing nodal rhythm occurring after normal sinus rhythm.

digitalized or the rhythm may be converted to sinus rhythm by DC counter-shock. The latter is preferable because of the improvement in cardiac output.

Persisting controversies

- Usefulness of the atrial pacing wire as a lead for atrial electrogram in the diagnosis of supraventricular arrhythmia.
- DC defibrillation after digoxin therapy.
- The role and value of newer drugs such as verapamil in the treatment of supraventricular arrhythmias.

Ventricular arrhythmias

These abnormalities arise from irritable ventricular myocardium. They are inefficient and cause a diminished cardiac output. More importantly, the abnormal rhythm is very unstable and without warning ventricular fibrillation may follow. The early detection and treatment of ventricular arrhythmia is one of the most important features of the care of cardiothoracic patients. The ventricular extrasystole is the most common manifestation of an irritable ventricle. On the ECG it causes a wide, slurred QRS complex of a totally different shape to the normal QRS (Fig. 12.6). Ventricular tachycardia is regular in rhythm. Irregular, slurred QRS complications are usually due to atrial fibrillation causing a rate-induced bundle branch block.

Causes of ventricular arrhythmias (Table 12.2)

At first, the ventricular extrasystole may occur randomly, during the normal cardiac cycle. Progression may happen in one of two ways. First, the ventricular extrasystoles become more and more frequent and eventually ventricular tachycardia with no effective cardiac output occurs (Fig. 12.7). Second, the extrasystole may occur just as repolarization following a previously normal ventricular contraction is completed. The result of this is

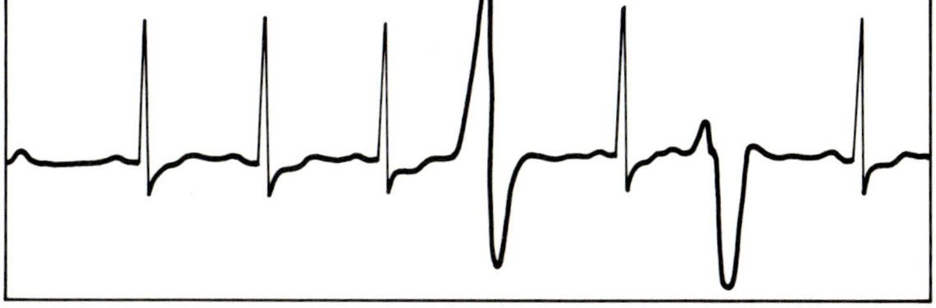

Figure 12.6
ECG showing multifocal ventricular ectopic beats.

Table 12.2
Causes of ventricular arrhythmias.

1 Myocardial damage
   (a) Temporary – as after cardiac surgery
   (b) Permanent – as after a myocardial infarction
2 Electrolyte abnormalities
   (a) Hypokalaemia
   (b) Hypercalcaemia
3 Hypoxia
4 Acidosis
5 Drugs
   (a) Adrenaline and other catecholamines
   (b) Digoxin

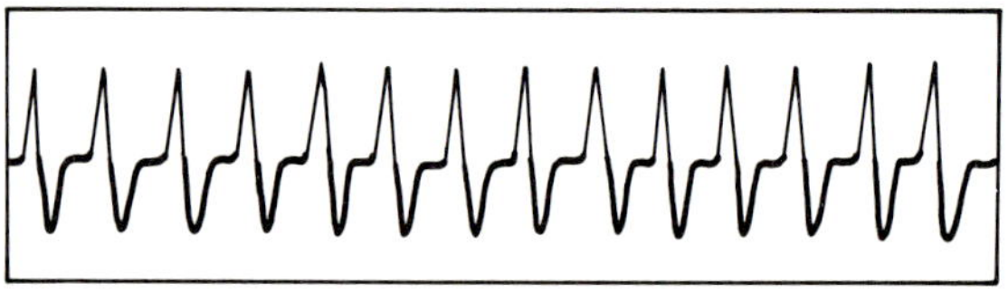

Figure 12.7
ECG showing ventricular tachycardia.

ventricular fibrillation and obviously no cardiac output. Ventricular extrasystoles thus have ominous significance and require treatment as soon as they are seen on the ECG. Several simple steps may be effective. Acidosis should be corrected and hypoxia reversed. The rate of infusion of catecholamines should be reduced or stopped.

One of the most important developments in cardiac surgery was the realization that the level of the serum potassium was important in the causation and prevention of ventricular arrhythmias. Studies showed that the maintenance of the serum potassium at around 5 mmol/l abolished most ventricular arrhythmias. Since the level of potassium in the serum changes very rapidly in cardiac surgery, and especially during cardiopulmonary bypass, frequent estimations of the serum potassium must be made. During bypass, the measurements are made every 30 minutes and after bypass every four hours. Potassium is infused intravenously to maintain a level of around 5.0 mmol/l. The amount of potassium needed will depend on the size of the patient, the level measured and importantly on the urine output. If ventricular arrhythmias occur when the level of potassium is unknown, then 2 mmol intravenously will often abolish them temporarily. Extensive clinical experience all over the world has confirmed the importance of the level of the serum potassium in the prevention of ventricular arrhythmias and the validity of the observation to other disciplines than cardiothoracic surgery is now accepted.

If ventricular arrhythmias persist in spite of a satisfactory serum potassium level, some drug treatment is indicated. Lignocaine, given first as a bolus of 1 mg/kg body weight and then as an infusion of the 0.1% solution, is effective. If lignocaine fails, there is severe myocardial damage and other drugs are less likely to be effective. On rare occasions, the arrhythmia may only respond to excision of a damaged area.

Summary Ventricular arrhythmias are caused by myocardial damage or by variations in the internal environment of the body. Some myocardial damage is clearly preventable at the time of surgery. When ventricular arrhythmias do happen, however, treatment of metabolic abnormalities should be the first priority. Attention is drawn to the importance of the serum potassium level. Only when this is corrected should antiarrhythmic drugs such as lignocaine be employed.

Persisting controversies

- The use of a small dose of potassium chloride to abolish ventricular arrhythmias.
- The role of drugs such as bretylium in the management of ventricular arrhythmia.

Conclusions

The cardiothoracic surgeon must become expert in the management of arrhythmia in cardiothoracic patients. The urgency of treatment means that there is often no time to call in a physician. In addition, the need for rapid treatment may not be appreciated by the non-surgeon. Diagnosis is made by an interpretation of the ECG and the surgeon must develop this skill. Prevention of myocardial damage during surgery will reduce the incidence of arrhythmia. When the disturbances do arise, however, the first priority must be to correct the disorders of physiology which may be the causative factors. Only after that stage should drugs be used.

Complications of Cardiac Pacing

The cardiac output falls to extremely low levels when the ventricles contract at less than 40 times per minute. The patient usually complains of symptoms which reflect inadequate cerebral perfusion. Periods of unconsciousness (Stokes–Adams attacks) may occur, but many patients will have less clear-cut symptoms such as attacks of giddiness or confusion. Since there are many causes of such symptoms, particularly in the elderly, and because the ventricular bradycardia may be transient and intermittent, the abnormality may be missed. The use of 24-hour monitoring of the electrocardiograph in the ambulant patient has detected a large number of such patients. As a result, the use of electrical cardiac pacemakers to maintain or increase the ventricular rate has increased enormously in the last few years and there is likely to be a further growth in the future.

Electrical pacemakers are in two distinct groups: first are the temporary systems used after surgery and after myocardial infarction, and second, totally implantable 'permanent' systems used in chronic rhythm problems.

Temporary cardiac pacing

The pacemaker is bulky and external to the patient. The electrical connection to the myocardium is achieved by conduction leads which enter the body either through a peripheral vein, if an endocardial site of stimulation is used, or by means of a chest incision for stimulation of the epicardium.

Endocardial temporary pacing of the ventricles is common in the treatment of temporary heart block occurring after myocardial infarction. The endocardial lead is passed via the venous system to the right ventricle where its active tip is jammed into the trabeculae. There are specific complications to the use of an endocardial pacing lead, whether it is temporary or permanent, and these are discussed below. The duration of pacing using an externally emerging lead, however, is obviously limited: sooner or later, contamination of the pacing wire will occur and thereafter systemic infection will inevitably follow. A temporary endocardial lead should be changed for a permanent system after seven to ten days should the need for pacing persist.

Temporary epicardial pacing is commonly used after cardiac surgery. Indeed, many prudent surgeons attach ventricular and perhaps even atrial pacing wires after every cardiac operation. Temporary disturbances of rhythm are common and unpredictable after cardiac surgery and the need for pacing may arise unexpectedly and abruptly. If no epicardial temporary wires are present, a damaging delay may occur.

Several surgical suture manufacturers make temporary epicardial pacing leads. They are made of stainless steel, each end having an atraumatic needle and all but the terminal few centimetres of the wire electrically insulated. Several superficial bites of the epicardium will achieve electrical contact and the wire may be held temporarily in place by a simple single plain catgut suture. The other end of the wire is brought through the chest wall and secured. When the time during which pacing may be needed has passed, simple traction will achieve removal of the wire.

Another advantage of placing epicardial wires at the time of surgery is that they are available should the need for an electrogram (i.e. an electrocardiogram recorded directly from the myocardium) arise during the diagnosis of an an unusual arrhythmia.

Complications of temporary cardiac pacing

Infection. The site at which the temporary leads emerge from the body will always be a channel by which infection may occur. Scrupulous asepsis should be employed in the insertion of a transvenous pacing lead and the leads should be covered by a sterile dressing and inspected daily. Should inflammation occur in the insertion site, then the lead will need removing forthwith, even if this means the insertion of another pacing lead at a different site.

Increasing pacing threshold. Temporary epicardial leads will begin to show an increasing threshold at which the ventricles may become stimulated within a few days, and within 14 to 21 days the pacing threshold may be beyond the capacity of the external pacemaker. Fortunately, most patients needing temporary pacing after cardiac surgery will have recovered normal rhythm by this stage. The remaining few patients who need pacing at around 10 to 14 days after operation should have a permanent system inserted.

Permanent cardiac pacing

The pacing system, i.e. the pulse generator and the conducting wire, is placed entirely within the patient's body. This technique has been made possible by the development of very small generators with a long life – nowadays upwards of ten years – but battery failure within the generator will need a second operation to replace the generator.

Most permanent pacing systems are now inserted by cardiologists with special interests in cardiac electrophysiology. Endocardial leads are used and connected to a generator inserted in the chest wall. Permanent epicardial systems demand some form of thoracotomy for their insertion and are relatively rarely used, and usually only after a failed attempt at placing an endocardial system.

Complications common to all permanent pacing systems

Infection The pacing system acts as a foreign body and, as in the case of cardiac valvular prostheses, normally non-pathogenic organisms may cause troublesome infection around the system. Once infection has become established, only removal of the entire system is effective in its treatment.

Prevention is never completely effective, but careful asepsis and handling of tissues during the insertion of the pacing system is essential. Most cardiologists will cover the period of insertion with prophylactic antibiotics for at least three days.

The diagnosis of infection in a pacing system may be very easy or exceptionally difficult. Part of the difficulty lies in the length of time after insertion during which infection may occur. Any infection up to one year after the operation should be assumed to be due to operative contamination. The discharge of pus after a period of wound inflammation is easily diagnosed, but the infection may be much more indolent and show itself by malaise and pain around the pacemaker box. There may be an accumulation of serous fluid in the pacemaker pocket leading to swelling and a loss of contact of the indifferent plate. The only effective treatment is to remove the entire pacing system. This is, however, not always possible because of the firm adherence of the myocardial end of the pacing lead within the heart. If prolonged traction fails to remove all the pacing wire, the wire should be cut short and, after the bare end has been insulated, allowed to retract away from the pacing box site. If endocarditis or persistent infection follows this limited procedure, then removal of the whole wire is essential – even if this means a thoracotomy. Some of the newer techniques of the interventional radiologist may help.

Pain and muscle twitching around the pacing box

This is a common complication but usually passes within a few days. If the symptom persists for more than a few weeks, however, the pacing box should be resited, preferably with the indifferent plate on the pacing box lying in contact with non-muscular tissue.

Necrosis and ulceration of the skin overlying the pacing box

This complication arises as a result of poor technique leading to ischaemia of the skin overlying the device. This may be due to the operator placing the pacing box too superficially or due to the skin being under tension when the wound is closed. Once necrosis occurs, the pacing box begins to protrude. Refashioning the wound is usually of no help for more than a few days and the pacemaker should be changed and resited. Sometimes, infection of the entire system will follow.

Specific complications of endocardial systems

Displacement of the pacing wire

In some patients, the pacing system works well for a short period after which the cardiac end of the wire displaces and the system fails. This complication seems to happen most frequently in short, squat patients especially if the heart lies horizontally.

The problem is prevented by the initial operator ensuring that the pacing wire tip impacts at the apex of the right ventricle or close to this area on the diaphragmatic wall. Once displacement has occurred, repositioning or changing the lead should be tried, possibly with a lead with a helical or 'screw-in' tip. If this fails, an epicardial lead is indicated.

Perforation of the right ventricle

Passage of the pacing wire tip through the thickness of the right ventricular free wall may be more common than thought or admitted. Haemorrhagic pericardial fluid is often found at subsequent surgery after a 'failed' endocardial pacemaker. Severe haemorrhage leading to tamponade is less common (four times out of 980 cases). When it does occur, the offending wire should be left in place and an emergency left anterior thoracotomy performed, if necessary in the pacing laboratory or catheter room. A buttressed horizontal mattress suture will control the laceration, but the main priority is to relieve tamponade.

Specific complications of epicardial systems

Epicardial pacing needs some form of thoracotomy in order to attach the pacing wire to the ventricular myocardium. Left anterior thoracotomy through the fifth intercostal space affords good exposure of the ventricles, but it is possible to insert a pacing electrode via an epigastric incision which continued extraperitoneally allows the diaphragm and diaphragmatic pericardium to be opened. The access is rather limited and there is not much choice over siting the electrode position. In addition, this epigastric exposure can be hazardous in the presence of adhesions in the pericardium. For most purposes, a left anterior thoracotomy is easier and quicker, and gives the surgeon more options over electrode siting.

Nearly all surgeons use some form of helical 'screw-in' electrode for epicardial pacing. If a site devoid of fat is chosen, a low pacing threshold is easily obtained and this threshold remains low over the years that follow. The prudent surgeon will, however, arrange for competent technical help in the operating theatre so that the pacing and sensing threshold can be measured before the chest is closed.

Complications

1 *High pacing threshold* (see above).
2 *Migration of the pacemaker box.* This is more common than when the box is inserted over pectoralis major. The box should be sited externally to the muscles of the abdominal wall. Pacing boxes placed deeper than this can erode into the peritoneal cavity. Again, the indifferent plate of the box should not lie in contact with muscle.

Summary

Cardiac pacing systems may be temporary or permanent. After surgery, it is common to insert epicardial wires to allow pacing externally if it should be required. All pacing systems may become infected and then only removal of the entire system will cure the infection. Prevention of infection is therefore crucial.

Most permanent systems are endocardial and implanted by cardiologists. The surgeon will only be asked to deal with difficult or failed cases. In these, an epicardial 'screw-in' electrode inserted at left thoracotomy is safe and reliable.

Persisting controversies

- Routine placement of epicardial wires at the time of cardiac surgery.
- The indications for atrial pacing.
- The best surgical approach for the insertion of permanent epicardial systems.

Conclusion

Electrical pacing of the heart is a sophisticated branch of cardiology and the indications for and choice of pacemakers must remain outside the responsibility of the surgeon. Most pacing systems will be successfully inserted by physicians using the endocardial route. The surgeon will be involved with complications which arise, however, and will also insert epicardial systems. A close relationship with the electrophysiologist is therefore essential.

Further reading

Bennett, D.H. (1981) *Cardiac Arrhythmias: Practical Notes on Interpretation and Treatment.* Bristol: John Wright and Sons.

Lockey, E., Longmore, D.B., Ross, D.N. & Sturridge, M.F. (1966) Potassium and open heart surgery. *Lancet, i,* 671.

Waldo, A.L. & Kaiser, G. (1973) Electrophysiological considerations for the cardiac surgical patient. In: *Preoperative, Operative and Postoperative Care of the Cardiac Surgical Patient,* ed. R.S. Litwak & R. Juanado. New York: Intercontinental Medical Book Corporation.

Waldo, A.L., Maclean, W.A.H., Cooper, T., Kouchokos, N.T. & Karp, R.B. (1978) The use of placed epicardial atrial wire electrodes for the diagnosis and treatment of cardiac arrhythmias following open heart surgery. *J. Thorac. Cardiovasc. Surg., 76,* 500.

Index

Principle references are indicated by **bold** type.